14375

636/SAM

A COLOUR ATLAS OF
LIVESTOCK BREEDS

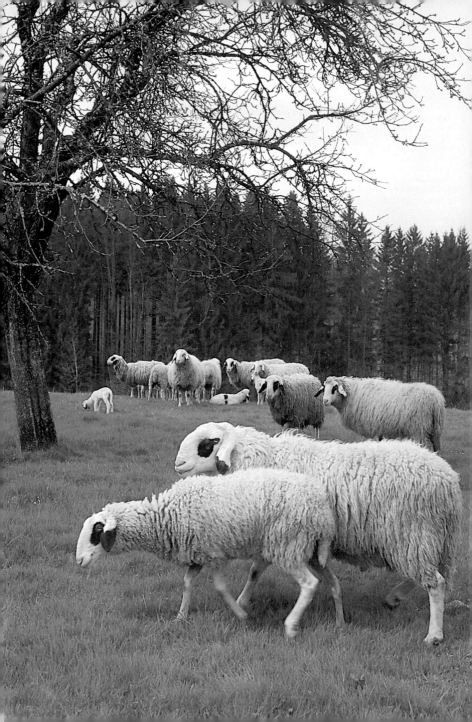

A Colour Atlas of

Livestock Breeds

220 breeds in words and pictures

Hans Hinrich Sambraus

Translated by Pam Chatterley

Wolfe Publishing Ltd

Cover photographs:

Piétrain pig (top left).
Carinthian spectacled sheep (top right).
Brown cow (lower left).
South German carthorse (lower right).

Frontispiece

Carinthian spectacled sheep.

Authorised translation of the 3rd German language edition 'Atlas der
Nutztierrassen' by H.H. Sambraus, 1989
Published by Verlag Eugen Ulmer, Stuttgart, Germany, 1989

Copyright © Eugen Ulmer GmbH&Co., 1989
Copyright © English language, Wolfe Publishing Ltd, 1992

Published by Wolfe Publishing Ltd, 1992
Printed in Germany
ISBN 0 7234 1891 8

A CIP catalogue record for this book is available from the British Library.

For full details of all Wolfe titles, please write to
Wolfe Publishing Ltd, 2–16 Torrington Place, London WC1E 7LT,
England.

Preface

Our livestock species are dominated by several breeds. These are described in all the textbooks, and illustrated in many. The numerous other breeds – remnants of old land races, exotics or breeds that have come from other countries and have not become widely distributed – are scarcely mentioned. But it is precisely these that provide patches of colour in our pastoral culture; they are a part of many landscapes, they help to utilise marginal land, and they form the livelihood of a number of people. The prime purpose of this book is to make us familiar with these breeds, to demonstrate their usefulness, and to highlight their importance as a cultural asset.

I have attempted to cover the breeds of hooved animals comprehensively, but it is in the nature of the task that this is not entirely possible. To a greater extent than in earlier times, there is currently a state of flux: new breeds are being added, special colour variations are deemed to be new breeds, and other breeds are no longer kept. I have covered poultry and rabbits only as *species*. Nevertheless, some breeds are shown to give an impression of the amazing variety of these species, but it would be outside the scope of this book to illustrate and describe all the breeds. For these, I refer the interested reader to the numerous well-illustrated specialised works, some of which are published by the breed associations.

The book is intended for animal breeders, veterinary surgeons and zoologists, as well as for those studying these subjects. It is often the zoologists who are familiar with the most extravagant physiological mechanisms or the most subtle genetic relationships, but who cannot differentiate or classify the breeds. This book will also make it possible for any interested lay person, who observes the countryside with an alert mind, to recognise the individual breeds. It is my aim, in an age when everything is standardised, to demonstrate the variety and rich diversity of our domestic animals, in the hope that they will be preserved. Fröhlich and Schwarzenecker wrote in 1926: 'The cultural standing of countries can be determined from the multiplicity of their types of horses: the more uniform they are, the lower is the culture.' Why should this be restricted to horses?

I have to thank many people who have given me information on individual breeds, above all Mrs Evelyn Simak, who in particular has a wonderful knowledge of our horse breeds. I would also like to thank all the breeders and breed associations which, without exception, were ready to give information, to show their animals with great patience, and to provide literature or illustrations which otherwise would have been difficult to obtain.

I would like to thank Mrs Edda Beutler for her thorough and constructive reading of the manuscript. Mrs Ingeborg Ulmer was exceedingly helpful in her careful and knowledgeable reading of the manuscript. I am grateful to Verlag Eugen Ulmer for the generous production of the book and for not insisting on originally agreed aspects, but accepting my wishes for alterations and additions.

Hans Hinrich Sambraus

Preface to the second and third editions

In the three years since it appeared, the atlas has found an unexpectedly wide readership. This fact together with the numerous favourable reviews of the book have confirmed that both the illustrations and the necessarily brief text are sufficiently comprehensive.

However, there can hardly be a book published that does not seem to require improvement when reviewed after a period of time. Suggestions came from many quarters. I am very much obliged to Mr Ludwig Bauer of Eichstätt, who gave me the benefit of his extensive experience and expert knowledge for the descriptions of the Soviet horse breeds. The second edition provided the opportunity to produce not only an improved, but also an enlarged edition. The book aims to illustrate the wealth of forms of the domesticated varieties. The breeds that occur in the German-speaking countries are only a small part of the total existing variety. For this reason, some breeds from other countries are included because they are involved in the crossing and improvement of breeds, or to arouse or maintain interest in them.

The second edition very quickly became out of print. It thus became possible to eliminate some errors which had persisted from the first edition. I am very grateful to observant readers for pointing them out. Some illustrations have been replaced with more impressive ones. I hope that these improvements help to bring the book a bit closer to its aim of facilitating the identification of livestock breeds.

Hans Hinrich Sambraus

Dedication

For Catherine and Daniel

Contents

Introduction

The meaning of livestock

By domestic animals we mean those which are in the care of people and are isolated from animals of the same species living in the wild. Mutations and intentional selection of certain individuals for breeding have resulted in domestic animals having different physical and physiological characteristics, capabilities and behaviour patterns from their wild ancestors. These characteristics are hereditary. The term 'domestic animal' is equivalent to 'domesticated animal'.

Wild animals that have been caught and tamed are not domestic animals, even if they have been in human hands for generations, in that they do not differ from the initial form in hereditary characteristics. Feral animals are not domestic animals in the true sense as they are not in the care of humans and are not subject to intentional selection. They do differ from wild animals in hereditary features, however.

Within the scope of domesticated animals, agricultural livestock are those species whose products are eaten or processed and which are put to work by man. It is difficult to classify wild animals that are kept in human care. In so far as they represent a real commercial operation in agriculture – such as in recent times the fallow deer – it is necessary to designate them as agricultural livestock. This does not apply to the whole species, however.

Advanced human cultures would be unthinkable without livestock. Man would not have been capable of developing significant cultures centuries ago, the remains of which we marvel at today, nor would we be in a position to maintain our civilisation today. Occasional attempts at intensive husbandry of wild populations do indeed lead to better utilisation of the areas concerned. The result may be improved nutrition of the population and reliable stocks, as more meat is available. But it is in no way possible to provide for the nutritional needs of the whole of humanity in this way.

Domestic animals are utilised in many ways. Consider, first of all, human food supply. We eat meat and eggs, drink milk and consume many types of milk products, such as butter, cheese and yogurt. Many races consider livestock to be status symbols and do not slaughter them, but nevertheless obtain blood from them for consumption and thus meet part of the inevitable need for animal protein.

Animal organs and substances are also processed into many types of products: wool for fabrics and carpets, skins for fleeces and leather which are used for clothing and footwear, and hair which is used for mattresses, paint brushes or tent fabrics. Horns are made into jewellery, utensils and musical instruments. Hollow organs, such as the stomach, intestines and bladder serve as cases for sausage meat or cheese. Whole skins serve as containers for storing and transporting water and wine. Animal products are used in medicine: as skin substitute, for stitching material after operations or animal charcoal for treating certain digestive problems. Hormones are obtained from endocrine glands. Other products made from animal organs are soap, glue, candles, strings for musical instruments and hairs for the bows of string instruments. As the covers of drums and tambourines, animal products form the basis of artistic creation or improve the quality of life.

The dung from livestock maintains the fertility of agricultural land. Dried dung is burnt in areas of the world where fuel is scarce. It serves not just to provide heat, but is also used for cooking. It was not so long ago that cattle dung was used in this way on the Hallig islands off the North Sea coast.

In our present state of motorisation it is easy to forget that throughout almost all of human history domestic animals used for work, transport and riding made human civilisation possible. Horses, cattle, buffalo and camels were put before the plough; they operated water wheels and assisted in threshing. Horses, donkeys and cattle pulled carts and thus facilitated extensive trade. Horses pulled coaches and thus increased the pleasure of a holiday or emphasised the dignity of a potentate. Horses, mules, camels and llamas crossed inhospitable mountain ranges carrying loads and traversed hostile deserts. Only in this way was it possible to settle faraway areas and later to maintain contact with the rest of the world. North American Indians were only able to penetrate into the prairie from the border territories to hunt bison because they possessed horses – indirectly via white people – and could ride. Only thus was it possible for them to leave dry areas at suitable intervals to return to water. Goods could be exchanged, skills could be acquired, and messages could be sent quickly. Domestic animals were also used to wage wars, be it to carry soldiers or to pull the materials necessary for war. They made the migration of peoples possible, and also enabled peoples to flee quickly in times of emergency.

Furthermore, we use animals in situations where our own senses are inadequate. This applies not only to hunting, where the dog (which will not be dealt with further here) with its superior sense of smell is an invaluable assistant to man. Pigs smell truffles in the earth and uproot them. It is fabled that geese have warned of raiders with their cackling. Guinea fowl alert other livestock to predators and thus protect the owner from commercial loss.

12

An important reason for breeding was often to obtain divergent forms and different capabilities. Dwarf forms, many types of physical deformity, hairlessness, special plumage or behaviour stereotypes due to hereditary brain anomalies were so valued in several areas of the world that the original purpose has lost its importance. Furthermore, among the different species there are various breeds in which an ability to run fast (horse, dog) or belligerence (cattle, dog, hen, goose, fish) is desired.

The coexistence of livestock and man is regarded as symbiotic, meaning that they both derive benefit from the association. This is doubtless true and until recently applied without qualification: man and livestock lived under the same roof, and even to a certain extent in the same room, with advantages and disadvantages for both. Today the advantages of this symbiosis are very unequally divided between man and animal. Livestock provide us with affluence and pleasure. In intensive rearing we grant them little more than survival, and that only for egotistical reasons. Keeping animals has become animal production, in English-speaking countries even 'animal industries'. Dead animals have become 'losses', which only attract attention because they may place the commercial viability of the holding in question. We should become more conscious that animals can suffer and that livestock too are individual beings that can enrich human life.

Of the larger livestock mammals occurring in central Europe, cattle and sheep are the most numerous in the world with a population of over 1 billion (**Table 1**). In third place is the pig at almost 800 million, followed by the goat. The solid-hoofed ungulates are numerically of less importance. All cloven-hoofed animals have greatly increased in numbers world-wide in the past 50 years, while the number of solid-hoofed ungulates has fallen during this time. The donkey is an exception, being most numerous in the 1960s.

The extent of livestock husbandry in different regions and continents is very variable. In this context, however, the difference in size of the

Table 1. World populations of various livestock animals (in millions).

Animal species	1937–39	1947–52	1967/68	1985
Cattle	615.0	764.3	1,099.4	1,268,934
Sheep	635.0	778.4	1,063.6	1,121,993
Goats	238.4	287.1	380.6	459,960
Pigs	260.0	295.7	605.2	791,471
Horses	73.0	75.8	66.0	64,631
Donkeys	33.8	36.5	42.5	40,509
Mules/hinnies	20.0	14.8	14.9	14,892

Source: FAO Production Yearbooks.

regions should not be forgotten. If the figures were related to units of surface area or human population densities, the relationships would doubtless be different. It can be seen that the greatest numbers of all animal species, apart from the horse, are in Asia. Horses are most common in North America.

When animal populations in individual countries are compared, it is not surprising to find that solid-hoofed ungulates and pigs are most numerous in the enormous People's Republic of China. India has the most cattle, the meat for religious reasons generally not being used commercially. Instead, the goat is kept because the favourable climatic and ecological conditions in India are suited to it. In Europe, each species of livestock is most widely distributed in a different country.

Domestication

Today almost everyone agrees that each domesticated animal species is descended from only one wild animal species. It is true that domesticated forms with very different appearances, which also have different names (dromedary/Bactrian camel, llama/alpaca, European cattle/zebu), are sometimes clearly descended from the same wild form. This fact was scarcely realised for a long time, although the laws of heredity and the principles of mutation and selection apply equally to the domestic animal population. But in each species there were breeds or individuals which differed considerably in size, colouring, hair structure and proportions of parts of the body. **Table 2** shows the derivation of domesticated forms from wild forms. Detailed studies of behaviour, physique and physiological reactions of domestic animal breeds in conjunction with consideration of

Table 2. Ancestry of livestock mammals kept in central Europe (details for poultry are in the relevant sections).

Domestic animal	Non-domesticated ancestor	
	Common name	Latin name
Cow	Aurochs	*Bos primigenius*
Domestic buffalo	Water buffalo	*Bubalus arnee*
Domestic yak	Wild yak	*Bos mutus*
Sheep	Mouflon	*Ovis ammon*
Goat	Bezoar goat	*Capra aegagrus*
Pig	Wild boar	*Sus scrofa*
Horse	Przewalski's horse	*Equus przewalskii*
Donkey	Wild donkey	*Equus africanus*
Rabbit	Wild rabbit	*Oryctolagus cuniculus*

the region of earliest domestication enable one to determine the sub-species of the wild form from which the domesticated form developed.

A biological prerequisite for the domestication of a species is the possibility of imprinting. Imprinting occurs when young animals are separated from their own kind shortly after birth and are reared by another species, in particular by man. Such individuals later feel that they belong to the species on which they have imprinted. If they have imprinted on humans, the result is that they do not fear people but want contact with them. They also prefer to direct their aggression and mating attempts at people (1). In contrast, they fear their own species.

A prerequisite for domestication by man is a need for the products and abilities of the animal species concerned. It is assumed that tame animals will help man to survive times of need. They should not, however, be species that could prove dangerous to man because of their size, strength and aggression. They should not be species that compete with man for the same food, or at least they should be content to live in captivity on man's food waste, as for example, the pig. Finally, tamed wild animals must be prevented from escaping by means of tethering, fencing or walls. Later, when the domesticated form differs from its wild forebears in ways man wishes, it must be prevented from mating with this original type so that the inbred advantages are not lost. This assumes a lengthy process of selection over many generations. Domestication therefore brings advantages for man, but also disadvantages in the continuous need for care of the animals.

It is very probable that the original reasons for the domestication of individual species differ from today's uses. The productivity of the wild form differed considerably from that of the domesticated animals. The wild form of sheep, goats and guanaco, for example, had no wool. The Bankiva hen lays few eggs, which would certainly not warrant keeping it in captivity all year. The milk production of female wild mammals is only sufficient to feed their own young. Man could not have guessed that productivity would develop so much during the process of domestication (Herre and Röhrs, 1973). It is assumed that individual species (dog, pig) associated with man of their own accord and lived on his food scraps. Other animals may have served initially as sacrifices in cult activities (Nachtsheim, 1936), with perhaps a certain stock of living animals being kept. These could have formed the starting point for domestication. It is assumed that arable farming started before cattle breeding. Arable farming demands a settled form of existence. Wild animals had to be kept away from the cultivated crops. If, however, they were still to serve as hunting prey, large distances would have to be covered to reach their habitat. It would therefore be better to keep them in enclosures and feed them on some of the cultivated crops.

Today there are about 20 species of mammal and about 10 species of bird world-wide that are used commercially. This does not include working animals and those kept for their fur, nor species like the guinea pig that were initially domesticated for meat, but now serve entirely different purposes. Sometimes certain other species are assumed to have been domesticated in earlier advanced cultures, and then later abandoned.

This assumption, which is based on early drawings, has not been confirmed by findings of bones, however. It is possible that the animals depicted were tamed wild animals.

The first animals were domesticated during the Neolithic period, i.e. the New Stone Age (2). This part of human history was a time during which significant advances were made, e.g. the cultivation of specific crops and the start of pottery making. We thus talk of the 'Neolithic revolution'. This term gives the mistaken impression that such changes occurred suddenly within a short period of time. However, this age occupied about a thousand years. Domestication of animals first took place where the wild forms occurred naturally.

There were certain centres of domestication. In large areas of the world no animal species were domesticated, although species existed there that seem eminently suitable for domestication and the people living there later obtained domestic animals from other areas. Presumably there was no domestication in regions where there was no fodder for domestic animals or where the climate or geographical conditions prevented the keeping of animals. In areas rich in game, it was unnecessary to domesticate the species occurring there as the population could obtain adequate food all the year round. Many human societies kept only dogs, which enjoyed a special status. Their meat was eaten only in certain situations and by certain peoples.

Return to the wild

From all species of livestock, groups of animals would escape from human care from time to time and become feral. By becoming feral we mean that from then on the animals were not subject to selection by man, only to natural selection. Above all, the term 'returning to the wild' means that the animals resemble wild animals in their behaviour and in their fear of man. This fear develops very quickly. Individuals of cultivated breeds in central Europe that had escaped, subsequently evaded a few unsuccessful pursuits, became widespread over great distances, and became nocturnal. Cows produced calves in the winter in the wilderness and reared them successfully. In Argentina, cattle which are kept extensively in semi-desert lands generally see human beings only once a day when they arrive by Jeep to check them. As soon as they see

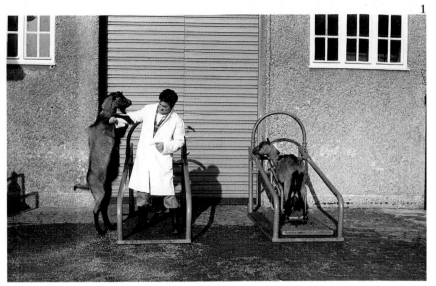

1   Mating attempt of a billy goat imprinted on humans.

people cows immediately summon their calves and flee into the bush. The notion that feral animals, in contrast to those in captivity, assume all the behaviour patterns of the original wild form, is mistaken. Domestic animals in human care retain all their original behaviour repertoire. No aspect of behaviour is lost by domestication; only the intensity and the frequency change. In the case of the feral animal, the behaviour patterns which seem to have been lost soon reappear in the presence of suitable trigger mechanisms among the considerably more varied environmental stimuli.

There are four reasons for domestic animals returning to the wild:

- They were left behind, centuries ago by seafarers on their voyages, to provide food for a future return visit.
- They escaped in thinly populated regions and could not be recaptured. In Australia there are herds of feral cattle which, over a period of time, have wandered hundreds of kilometres from the place of their escape. Only after a long time did they settle in a region that suited them.

Years BC	'Fertile Crescent'	Northern Greece	Central Europe	Ukraine	North America
12000			dog		
11500					
11000					
10500					
10000	dog				
9500					
9000	sheep				
8500					dog
8000				pig	
7500	sheep goat		dog		
7000	pig				
6500		sheep goat			
6000	cattle	goat cattle pig			
3500					
3000				horse	

2   The earliest evidence of domestic animals in various regions of the world (from Boessneck, 1983).

- They were left behind when isolated industrial areas (e.g., 'Death Valley' in the USA) or farms were abandoned for economic reasons or in times of drought.
- Domestic animals (dogs, cats) were deliberately released in areas where feral animals of other species had increased in number disproportionately and had become a danger to the rest of the animal world and the ecology. It was hoped, sometimes mistakenly, that the predators would decimate the harmful animals.

It can be assumed that the populations of feral domestic animals were originally land races. This means that the original form lived in an intemperate climate and was accustomed to withstanding the rigours of the weather and poor nourishment. Furthermore, such animals generally resemble the wild form in physique more than cultivated breeds, and differ greatly in shape, size, colouring and in their ability to adapt. Undoubtedly, natural selection affects feral populations and removes carriers of unsuitable genes. Nevertheless, there is still a considerable range of variation: this can be seen mainly in their coloration. In many populations that returned to the wild very early on, there is nearly the full range of colours and combinations of colours that occur in an animal species. It is different only when the initial form, the domestic animal, was homogeneous with respect to a characteristic. Chillingham cattle in the UK, which are known to have been subject to no artificial selection for centuries, are exclusively pure white. No colour similarity to the wild form has occurred. It is remarkable that feral animals may have colorations (e.g. dappling in feral donkeys in South Dakota) that rarely appear in the corresponding domestic animals. Presumably these mutations did not occur for the first time among the feral animals, but were already present in the original domesticated form. Dappling was very much admired by several peoples, and has thus persisted, for example, in mustangs, the feral horses of Spanish ancestry in North America.

Feral animals subject to natural selection thus bear only a slightly increased resemblance to the wild form. However, they sometimes demonstrate excellent adaptability to the habitat that they have acquired by chance, which at times surpasses that of the wild form: there are feral cattle on islands where it does not rain for most of the year. As there are no other sources of water, the animals meet their need for liquid by licking the dew from plants in the morning. Soay sheep, for example, go to the beach and eat very salty seaweed.

Sometimes feral animals are again taken into captivity and are then considered as a breed in the form found or after suitable selection. This applies to some North American horse breeds (e.g. Appaloosa) and also, for example, to the Texas Longhorn cattle. Today mustangs are captured mainly in the American north west and sold to buyers in other parts of the USA for several hundred dollars. Tamed mustangs, which may well become another separate breed, have long had a special name: broncos.

In the UK on the St. Kilda islands the Soay sheep, which became feral many centuries ago, has recently been taken into captivity again. It is a remarkably shy animal.

Diversity of breeds

By the word breed we mean a group of domesticated animals that resemble one another in essential morphological and physiological characteristics, and have a common breeding history. The dividing line between one breed and another is sometimes difficult to determine. If similar forms occur in neighbouring regions, there will, as a rule, be an exchange of breeding material. In this case, one can speak of different strains of *one* breed. If similar forms are separated geographically, and one does not derive from the other, they would be considered as different breeds. This still applies if there is an occasional exchange of blood. The question of how great the similarities must be in order to speak of one breed remains unanswered. Undoubtedly, German Friesian cattle, for example, differ from the Dutch. But they are similar compared with the North American Holstein Friesians, which are descended from them. The central European Friesians even resemble the original Freiburg black spotted cattle, to which they are not genetically related, more than the Holstein Friesians. Is there therefore a breed of German Friesians, or of the Friesians around the North Sea and the Baltic, or of European Friesians, or of Friesians in general?

There are greatly differing views on this. For example, a Jutland that is brought to the Federal Republic of Germany for breeding purposes is treated as a Schleswig carthorse there. This is only possible, however, because the two breeds are very similar. Indeed, a difference in one single gene is enough to move an individual from the breed of its parents into another breed, e.g. owing to the resultant different coloration.

For some time the word breed has often been replaced by the word population. This has not made definition any easier. So, population can mean anything from the animals of a breed society to the totality of all domesticated animals of a species. Furthermore, this term is largely synonymous with the term breed.

Breeds arise by the selection for breeding of individuals with specific characteristics, and by the exclusion from reproduction of those animals that do not have these characteristics (in the case of qualitative features) or in which they are not sufficiently marked (in the case of quantitative features). These features are very varied. They can be morphological as well as behavioural characteristics. Behind each behavioural characteristic there is bound to be a characteristic in the central nervous system, just as there is a physiological mechanism behind each product of the living animal (eggs, milk, wool). But the breeder cannot see this; he keeps to what he can identify.

Physical characteristics do not mean only the amount of meat or fat. There are features that improve the animal's ability to adapt to certain climatic conditions. Thick, long hair in breeds that are kept in harsh climates (e.g. Scottish Highland cattle), or sparse hair cover in the tropics (e.g. zebus, hairy sheep) increase tolerance to cold and heat respectively. The same applies to the occurrence of a skin which is large compared with the body size, with many folds or other marked skin organs, which serve to conduct heat away: zebus have a particularly marked dewlap and a very pendulous prepuce. Mamber goats possess extremely long ears (3). Horns are another feature of selection. Animals can be bred to be hornless or to have several horns (four-horned sheep and goats) or to have particularly long and extensive horns.

Having long horns or twice the original number of horns does not necessarily improve an animal's ability to fend off other animals in a fight. They are either a curiosity or serve to impress people and thus increase the prestige of the owner. Other characteristics have even less practical origins. This applies especially to coloration. Particularly well-marked animals often simply please the owner. In other cases it is considered that particularly good performance is associated with certain colorations. Even today, it is sometimes said in Allgäu that belted cattle (4), a variety of brown cattle, give a lot of milk.

Dark spotted bulls are said to have a strong desire to mate. The tendency to infer future performance from identifiable characteristics is understandable; it is generally the case, however, that there is little connection. Nevertheless, selection by such features has contributed to the formation of breeds. Uniformity in certain characteristics has often made it possible to recognise cross-breeds.

Sometimes the mating partners for an individual have been sought exclusively and over a long period within its own breed. We speak then of a 'closed studbook'. This is the case, for example, with the English thoroughbred or the Galloway. With many breeds, they are sometimes crossed with breeds similar in appearance, to maintain the characteristic features. This applies for example to the German riding horse and the Shagya.

Another reason for mating animals of different breeds is the modification of the breeding aim as a result of altered user expectations. The change from the fat pig to the meat pig and the breeding of larger sheep

3

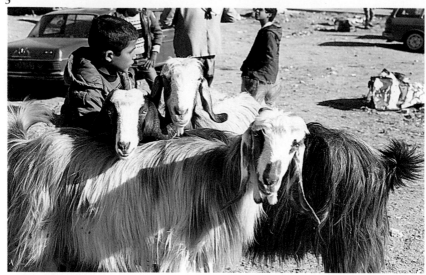

3 Mamber goat.

with better meat formation at the expense of the wool quality are examples of this process. It is true that the genetic variability of a breed is generally great enough to produce a modification from within itself, but this is a lengthier and more cumbersome process. In general, a breed suitable for cross-breeding is one which comes close to the new breeding target and which is similar in phenotype to the breed to be improved.

The reason for this is that the breeders do want to improve performance; but they are also attached to the breed they have raised in the past and want to maintain its essential features. This explains why the white-headed Herefords of North America have been crossed with the Simmental (spotted cattle), which also has a white head, to produce a larger frame. To improve the milk production of the Pinzgau and the spotted cattle in Austria and Switzerland, the Red Holstein was chosen, and not for instance the black and white Holstein Friesian.

The way cross-breeding is carried out depends on its purpose. The interbreeding is for refinement if sire animals of certain other breeds are occasionally crossed with the native breed. This method is used with several horse breeds. In this way, appearance and valuable characteristics as well as the existing compatibility with local conditions are retained.

In combination cross-breeding, at least two initial breeds are mated to produce a completely new type. The young in the next generations differ quite considerably, and intensive selection is necessary to achieve the

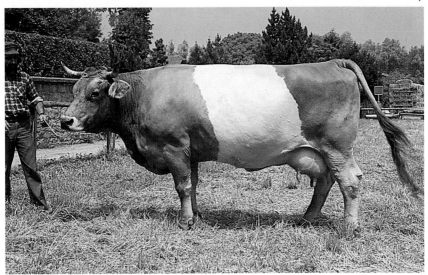

4 Belted cow.

desired aim. Many of the breeds we have today were produced in this way. Examples from the recent past include the aurochs retro-breed and the German Angus cattle.

In displacement cross-breeding, the female animals of a native breed are mated exclusively over several generations with an improving breed which has the required characteristics. As the genetic material of the local breed is halved with each successive generation, after six generations only 1.6% of the original genes are retained, or to put it another way: 98.4% of the gene material comes from the inbred breed. This means that the animals are almost identical to the inbred breed in appearance and performance. The inbred breed has displaced the initial breed. Such a displacement occurred with the pig as a result of the economic upturn in the then Federal Republic of Germany and the associated consumer expectations. The improved German land pig, which was of the fat pig type, was crossed with boars of Danish and Dutch ancestry to produce a meat pig with considerably less fat and a greater proportion of high-quality meat. This change of type was later recognised by changing the name of the breed. Often, cross-breeding is performed to achieve heterosis effects. Heterosis means that the descendants of the next generation will, on average, have better performance than their parents and, where possible, will surpass the best of the parents. When crossing two breeds, the animals resulting from the cross are not used for breeding, but are slaughtered. When crossing three breeds, a sow of breed A is covered by a boar of breed B. The female animals resulting from this mating are later covered by a boar of breed C and thus produce the end product for fattening.

Hybridising is a special form of cross-breeding. First, many breeds and lines are tested to determine which combination of 'matching lines' is the most suitable. Position effects are used in addition to heterosis effects. Hybrid breeding is only possible on a large scale and with many participants.

There were specific breeds that differed from one another soon after the start of domestication. Findings of bones and drawings show that even in Assyria and Babylonia, among the Ancient Egyptians and in the Roman Empire, there were different breeds of a species side by side, and that at certain times, various breeds were kept in different areas of the world. Such multiplicity is a result of different applications, adaptation to the local conditions, and the individual taste of owners or population groups. The geographical separation of two population groups (by islands, valleys, oases) contributes to this variety.

The expression 'race' or 'breed' has been used in animal breeding for several centuries. Originally it referred to the totality of animals of a species in a certain region, which, despite considerable variability in size, appearance or performance, differed to a certain extent in some features from the population of other regions. Variation within a reproduction community was even desired, in order to meet the different needs of the owners. It was not until the second half of the eighteenth century that clear ideas on breeding purpose and selection of animals that best met that aim corresponded to the development of breeds in our sense. Initially, inbreeding was often used to establish the breeding aim.

The breeds we have now are not so very old. Most arose during the nineteenth century or even at the start of this century. It is true that individual animals that resemble current breeds phenotypically occurred far earlier, as descriptions and drawings reveal. Deliberate and consistent breeding was a response to the increasing demand for animal products which resulted from industrialisation. The animal stock was improved partly by importing proven breeds, by cross-breeding with the native population, and by displacement. Also, the original variety of the stock had become reduced. The remaining breeds thus had a broader breeding basis.

In the nineteenth century there were 46 different named 'breeds' of cattle in Bavaria. Today, in many cases we would, without hesitation, group several of these different forms into one breed; they are in fact strains. Four strains alone resemble the Pinzgau in their colour. In addition to one principal coloration, several other colours were described for most breeds. The statement that Pinzgaus accounted for 20.5% of the cattle population in Upper Bavaria in 1883, but only 13.1% nine years later (Rasp, 1893), should not be taken to mean that nearly half of this breed had disappeared and been replaced by other cattle. The fact is that during this time displacement cross-breeding took place in the form of interbreeding with bulls of another breed (apparently Simmental) which changed the phenotype of the population. Some breeds were lost subsequently (e.g. the Triesdorf cattle), while others (e.g. Mainland as a strain of the Franken cattle) resembled in coloration those we have today from as early as the middle of the last century (5). It is true that those earlier breeds did not resemble their descendants, which we have today, either in weight or in type. It is worthy of note that development in the past hundred years has not been linear, as can be seen in DLG reports. This reflects the variability of the genetic material, as long as there is no crossing with other breeds. If, however, in the future there should be selection plateaux – promoted by the widespread use of only a few sires for artificial insemination – a breed will not be able to overcome this plateau on its own. This is one of the reasons why breeds which currently have only a few individuals, i.e. with a breed conformation that does not match the trend, should not be abandoned. It would not be unusual if characteristics were suddenly valued that had been previously over-looked, not recognised or regarded differently owing to certain user expectations. A livestock breed is a cultural asset that should not be destroyed any more than an old tree, a historic building or a work of art. There are already programmes aimed at preserving endangered old breeds. This can be done, among other things, by providing premiums for breeding, keeping and covering.

In several cases, nuclear herds have been set up in government establishments. In addition, semen and embryos are deep frozen as a gene reserve, and can be used if necessary. Often the old land races differ considerably in form and coloration from the standard and are thus particularly attractive, being shown in animal parks. Recently, action has been taken in various areas to make regionally endangered breeds accessible to the public on special farms.

Classification of breeds

The range of variation within breeds is generally greater than the differences between individuals within a species. In addition to common characteristics, there are many in which the individual animals within a breed differ. Occasionally, quite disparate individuals are required within quite homogeneous breeds. For example, it is not possible for a shepherd to count hundreds of sheep in broken countryside to find out whether

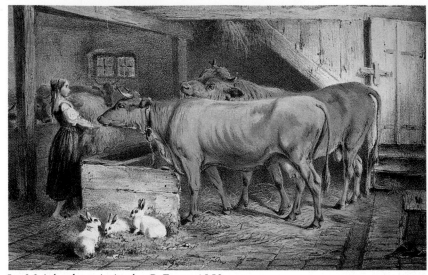

5   Mainlands: painting by G. Fraas, 1853.

some are missing. If, however, every fiftieth is black, it suffices to count these animals to check whether a large part of the flock is missing. In some regions, a pure-bred animal with different colouring is regarded as lucky; it is in no way despised. Therefore, it is not possible to provide a reliable key to classification as in zoology and botany. There is often some doubt when examining an individual animal. Classification is easier if several animals of one breed can be examined together. It is easier still if one knows what breeds occur in the region in question.

In the case of cattle, it is advisable to look at the colour first. There are single-colour black, red, brown, golden, grey and white breeds. Then there are spotted breeds, where white is combined with black as well as with red, brown and gold. There are also milky red and blue pigmentations. Another clue is the colour distribution. Is white or the colour predominant? Is the pigmentation or the white concentrated on certain body parts, or do unpigmented areas only appear as markings on certain parts of the body?

Some breeds have distinctively long hair and can thus be easily identified. The presence or absence of horns can only be used to classify cattle to a limited extent, as in many populations the animals are polled. In a large number of dehorned animals of a horn-bearing breed there will, however, generally be individual animals with residual horn stumps. When horns are present, the shape and length can facilitate classification of the animal.

The expert will immediately include the conformation of an animal, i.e. the overall appearance and the build, in the evaluation. Milking cattle breeds are generally wedge-shaped in build: the head is small, there is hardly any dewlap, the brisket is relatively shallow, and the hindquarters are particularly pronounced with a large udder. The lower line of the body descends from the mouth to the rear. In contrast, beef breeds have a deep brisket and a less pronounced udder; seen from the side, the body is therefore rectangular. Dual-purpose breeds have an appearance between these two extremes. Flat land races mostly have long legs. Other features that aid classification are large frames and muscle formation.

In the case of sheep, height and build can generally be judged easily, and when shorn, so can the type. It is more difficult with animals in full fleece because the wool can give the impression of a different type with greater muscling. The expert can assess the meat laid down by feeling the loin region.

As it is not usual to dehorn sheep, the few horned breeds are easily defined. A lay person could also make a rough assessment of the wool. It is at least possible to distinguish smooth and rough-woolled animals from merinos. Hairy sheep are often taken to be goats. They can, however, be differentiated from them externally by the longer, pendulous tail which has no ridges of hair on the sides, and also by the fact that they have fore-eye and inter-hoof glands.

Sheep breeds differ not only in the quality of the wool but also in the extent of wool growth. While in most breeds the tail bears wool, and in some breeds also the forehead and front of the legs, in other sheep breeds they are covered in hair.

The fleece is generally of one colour which may be white, yellowish (usually due to wool grease), reddish, brown, grey or black. Spotted sheep are rare. Either they occur as exceptions in certain breeds (e.g. Merino Landschaf), or the spotting is a characteristic of the breed (e.g. Jacob's sheep, which also has four horns, *see* p. 128). The colouring of the hair on the body parts without wool (head, legs, possibly tail) often differs from the colour of the wool. It can be white, reddish, brown or black. On these parts of the body, some breeds have dark spots or patches on a white background. Generally all parts of the body covered with hair have the same colour. An exception is the Rhön, in which the head is black but the legs are white. Additional criteria for determining the breed are ear position and shape of the bridge of the nose. A classification of the sheep breeds kept in German-speaking countries is given in **64**.

In the case of goats, the presence of horns can serve to distinguish the breeds, but with two qualifications. 1. Goats are sometimes also dehorned. 2. In Switzerland, some previously hornless breeds are now again being bred to have horns because of some loss of fertility associated with dehorning. Additional features that characterise breeds are the shape of the bridge of the nose, ear length, frame, and length of body hair.

Pigs can initially be categorised by type and frame. The fat pig type favoured in the past can be differentiated from the modern meat pig. East Asian breeds and those bred as experimental animals must be dealt with separately. They can be recognised easily by their small size. Fat pigs are mainly of large build, of medium length, with a deep breast and a voluminous belly. Their muscle formation is not apparent. Meat pigs are long with a small torso depth. The hams and shoulders are prominent. Colouring is an essential aid in classifying breeds. There are single-colour breeds – white, red, brown and black. Some breeds are mainly mono-coloured, but have some white markings (e.g. Berkshire). Other breeds have black patches, the main colour being white, grey or reddish. Belted pigs must be regarded as a special group in which the light-coloured belt always encircles the middle of the body. The pigmented parts of the body can be black or reddish brown.

Other body features that typify breeds are shown in **Table 3**.

In the case of horses, colour can only be used to a very limited extent to classify a breed. Unlike most other species of livestock, a breed is not generally linked to a particular colour. Exceptions are rare (e.g. Lipizzaner), and even there, different colours occur occasionally. Most breed societies permit all basic colours, and white markings may occur. Dappling, however, is not permitted. Apart from those breeds in which dappling is an essential prerequisite, it is rare for it to be bred in intentionally, in addition to other colour variations within a breed (e.g. Noriker).

Horse breeds vary enormously in size, so this characteristic can be used in breed classification. Up to a height at the withers of 148 cm they are classed as ponies, and above that height they are full-size horses. This parameter determines the breed group, but not the breed itself. To make things more difficult, some breeds have an average height of about this size, so some individuals must be classed as ponies, and others as horses (e.g. the Welsh Cob). Many ponies are not only small, but also match this breed group in type: they are stocky, muscular, round-bellied and relatively short-legged. Other breeds of pony largely resemble horses in

Table 3. Body features that typify breeds.

Head shape	Elongated (straight nose profile)
	Dished (curved nose profile)
Ear position	Upright ears
	Lop ears

their proportions. Among full-size horses, carthorses can easily be differentiated from other breeds. Carthorses are large-boned, muscular and have a relatively heavy head. Some breeds are also exceedingly large. Above all, carthorses have a 'split croup' (the muscles that form on the pelvis project either side of the rump bone), and a square body shape: the height of the back is the same as the length between the front and back legs. According to this criterion, the Friesian, for example is a heavy crossbreed (warmblood), and the Freiberger is a light carthorse. The remaining horse breeds are characterised by type and frame, as well as by, among other things, nose line, build, hair characteristics and relative leg length. The body shape of a crossbreed resembles a horizontal rectangle, and that of a thoroughbred resembles an upright rectangle.

Hens are classed by size into light, medium and heavy breeds as well as dwarf breeds. The Federation of German Poultry Breeders gives groupings according to physical features held in common (**Table 4**).

Dwarf hens, apart from the group of 'true dwarf hens', correspond to the six hen groups listed. In the case of hens, there are many marking types and colour strain groups. They are useful in further subdividing the groups listed and are contained in the *German Poultry Breed Standard* (N.N. 1984).

In the case of other species of poultry, the breeds are classified as with hens by size, type, shape, colour and markings. Details should be sought in specialised books.

Finally, it must not be forgotten that not all livestock can be definitely assigned to a specific breed on the basis of the information given. As shown in **Tables 5–7**, crossbreeds account for a considerable proportion of German livestock.

In the following breed descriptions, all dimensions are in centimetres, and weights are in kilograms, unless indicated otherwise.

Table 4. Grouping by common physical features.

Group	Common features
Fighting and related breeds	Red ear lobes, yellow pigmented legs
Asiatic breeds	Red ear lobes, short plumage, leg colour other than blue
Intermediate breeds	Type intermediate between Asiatic and Mediterranean
Mediterranean breeds	White ear discs, long plumage
Crested hens and related breeds	Modifications to skull and nose bones, white ear discs, long plumage, no yellow leg pigment
North-west European breeds	White ear discs, long plumage, no yellow leg pigment

Cattle

In the zoological system, the term 'cattle' is much broader than one would assume from observation of our domestic animals. Cattle form a sub-family within the large family of horned animals, which includes antelopes, sheep and goats. There are nine species of cattle, the buffalo being differentiated from the bisons and the true cattle. The horns, among other things, can serve as a definitive characteristic differentiating buffalo from true cattle. In buffalo, the horn cross-section is triangular, and in true cattle it is round. The genus of true cattle includes the aurochs, of which only domesticated forms survived. But some of the other true cattle were also domesticated (**Table 2**). All five species of true cattle (aurochs, gaur, banteng, kouprey and yak) can be interbred and crossed with bison, but as the male offspring are almost always infertile breeding can only continue with the females of the crossed animals. In North America, crossbreeds between European cattle breeds and bison (beefalo, cattalo) have some economic significance, as do crosses between zebu and yak on the fringes of the Himalayas.

Domestic cattle, which are descended from the aurochs, are subdivided into two large groups. One of these is the zebus, which occur primarily in Asia and Africa, and, since the last century, in South America and around the Gulf of Mexico. They can be recognised mainly by the hump in the breast or neck region, which is formed by an overdeveloped muscle. There is no overall term for the other breeds, those without humps, which we designate generally as cattle.

Sometimes one speaks of European cattle breeds, but native cattle without humps occur in Africa and East Asia as well.

The main use of cattle is for meat, milk and labour. These uses allow the classification of the approximately 450 cattle breeds in the world into breed groups. With some breeds, one of these three usage criteria is so dominant that they are called beef, dairy or draught breeds; these are so-called single-purpose breeds. Many cattle belong to dual-purpose breeds, where equal emphasis is placed on beef and milk production. If one of these uses is dominant, they are called beef-based or dairy-based dual-purpose breeds. The capacity for heavy work is no longer significant in western Europe, in North America and other high-technology regions, but it is still important on a world-wide scale. Good draught cattle are generally very muscular. It was therefore natural to develop draught breeds into beef breeds or beef-based dual-purpose breeds after motorisation, where they did not die out.

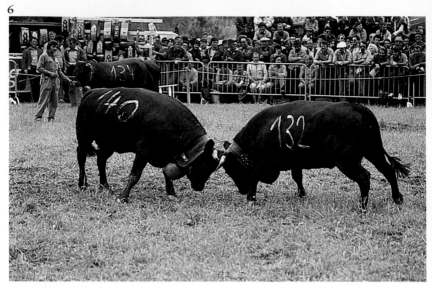

6   Fighting Eringers.

In addition to the highly-productive breeds, there are numerous land races which are mostly basically triple-purpose breeds, but are inferior to the types mentioned in each area of productivity. They are undemanding, hardy and tenacious. Often, the fact is overlooked that such animals can survive on considerably poorer nourishment than highly productive cattle, and in certain circumstances have advantages over the latter.

In addition to the main applications mentioned, there are numerous other uses which have moulded certain breeds, i.e. they are not merely subsidiary products. Cattle breeds in East Africa, which are kept for prestige reasons and are not slaughtered – only the milk and blood are used – have horns that are more than a metre long and enormously thick. Fighting cattle are kept on the Iberian peninsula, in Mexico and in southern France. Not only is the aggression of these animals with regard to people very marked, they are also very aggressive to one another. This means that avoidance distances between the animals are greater, so they cannot be stocked at such large densities as our cattle. Intensive rearing is therefore impossible. The very aggressive Eringers in Valais are allowed to fight one another. The fights are an important social event in the region (6), and a cow's success in fighting has a decisive effect on its commercial value.

Among the Hindus of India, the cow is a holy creature. According to legend, a cow once saved the life of the persecuted Krishna with its milk.

Krishna was the most popular and human incarnation of the universal god and world preserver Vishnu. Krishna's cow became the life-saving 'mother' of every Hindu believer, and so its meat may not be eaten. Anyone who does anything to a cow or is responsible for its death is guilty of a mortal sin that is worse than murdering a member of the upper caste, according to the orthodox religious morality of the Hindus.

In the German-speaking countries there are no native single-purpose breeds. In one case (Beef Shorthorn), they arrived in the last century, but most came in recent decades from other European countries (UK, France) or North America. Of those cattle breeds occurring in Germany, some have been very important for a long time (**Table 5**). These are dairy-based dual-purpose breeds such as Friesians, Spotted Cattle and Brown Cattle. The proportion of total production they represent has changed little in recent centuries; in general it has risen. Cattle numbers do not take account of breed. The figures are therefore based on the number of herd book animals recorded by the breed organisations. It is to be expected that the proportion of herd book animals will not be the same in all breeds, so there will be a certain amount of distortion in the figures.

Table 5. Total cattle population in the then Federal Republic of Germany by breed (only herd-book animals).

Breed	1951 %		1987 Number	1987 %	
German Friesian	34.3⎫		791,870	43.6⎫	
German Spotted	38.5⎬ 86.7		603,311	33.2⎬ 96.7	
German Brown	5.5⎪		185,160	10.2⎪	
German Red Friesian	8.4⎭		175,793	9.7⎭	
German Golden	7.7		26,078	1.4	
Angeln	1.1		13,592	0.7	
Vorderwälder ⎫			6,509	0.4	
Hinterwälder ⎭	0.8		576	0.0	
German Red	1.0		2,847	0.2	
Pinzgau	0.7		251	0.0	
Murnau-Werdenfels	0.2		100	0.0	
Jersey	0.0		2,883	0.2	
Charolais ⎫			3,306	0.2	
German Angus ⎪			1,490	0.1	
Limousin ⎬	0.4		789	0.0	
Galloway ⎭			858	0.0	
Scottish Highland Cattle	—		363	0.0	
Other breeds	1.4		272	0.0	
Total			1,816,048		

Source: Cattle production in the Federal Republic of Germany (German), 1985 Edition.

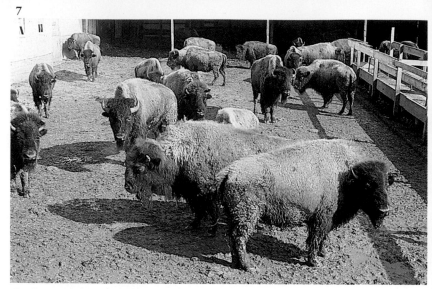

7   Intensive bison rearing.

The proportion of other native breeds has fallen. Only in recent years have attempts been made to preserve endangered breeds in gene banks with government support. There have been increases in beef breeds and land races which can be kept extensively. In Austria and Switzerland Spotted and Brown Cattle are the most frequent breeds. In both countries local breeds also occur to a lesser degree (**Tables 6** and **7**).

Table 6. Cattle in Austria 1985 (in thousands).

Breed	Number	%
Spotted	2,083	78.6
Brown	315	11.9
Pinzgau	97	3.7
Friesian	87	3.3
Grey	19	0.7
Others + crosses	49	1.8

Source: Zentrale AG of Austrian Cattle Breeders.

Table 7. Cattle in Switzerland 1983 (in thousands).

Breed	Number	%
Simmental Spotted	851	44.0
Brown	786	40.7
Black Spotted	229	11.9
Eringer	14	0.7
Others + crosses	52	2.7

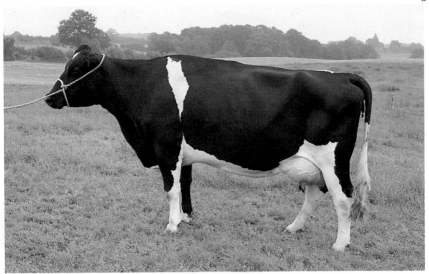

Friesian

Characteristics: Black and white. Black head with white markings. The eyes are always surrounded by pigmented skin. Owing to crossing with Holstein Friesians, the number of white areas of skin and white markings on the head have increased in recent years. The original type of German Friesian, which is hardly found nowadays, is of medium frame and medium muscling. The greater the proportion of Holstein Friesian blood that the animal has, the larger the frame, the longer the legs and the flatter the muscles. Horned, but polled animals are seen increasingly because of de-horning.

	Bull	*Cow*
Height at shoulder	152	140
Weight	1000–12000	600–700

Distribution: World-wide. Most numerous cattle breed in the world. German-speaking countries, particularly North Germany and East Germany.

Uses: Dairy-based dual-purpose breed. Annual milk yield of herd book cows on average 6100 kg (4.0% fat, 3.3% protein). Daily weight gain of fattening bulls on test stations is 1150 g.

Breed history: In the lowlands from Holland to Denmark, a cow whose high milk production was praised as long ago as the 16th century. In 1811 they were described as 'black and white, giving much milk and suitable for fattening and therefore used often for refining other German breeds'. The first herd book was produced in 1868. At about this time intensive breeding of 'Holstein Friesians' began in the USA. These were crossed with the European population, which was bred more as a dual-purpose type, to produce the modern type with extremely high milk production.

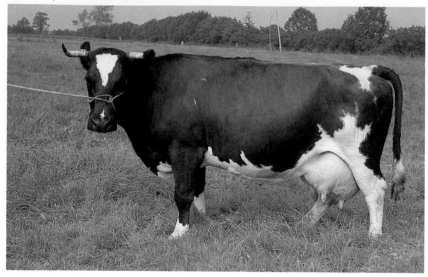

Red Friesian

Characteristics: Large. Dark red and white. The head is red with white markings. Until very recently a well-muscled cow of medium frame. By crossing with Red Holstein now taller and with flatter muscles. Horned. Now often dehorned.

	Bull	*Cow*
Height at shoulder	150	140
Weight	1100	700

Distribution: North and west Germany; fewer in the remaining area of the former Federal Republic. Similar forms with local names in other central European countries. As Red Holstein in North America.

Uses: Suitable for poorer locations. Good fodder utilisation. Dual-purpose cattle with equal emphasis on milk and beef production. Annual milk production is about 6000 kg (4.0% fat, 3.5% protein). Good milker. Young bulls achieve average daily weight gains of 1300 g. Carcase yield about 60%.

Breed history: Red and white animals have occurred as a minority among the cattle populations of the north German lowlands for a long time. From the start of the nineteenth century, they were bred in several regions as quite different strains, under the particular influence of the Shorthorn. In 1934 all German breeding areas were united. In North America the Red Holstein population was built up from the red and white animals occurring occasionally among the Holstein Friesians. Introduction of appropriate genetic material into the German Red Friesian breed allowed milk production to be increased with a subsequent change in the type and a reduction in muscle. The same occurred in other brown-spotted breeds, e.g. the Swiss Simmental and the Austrian Pinzgau.

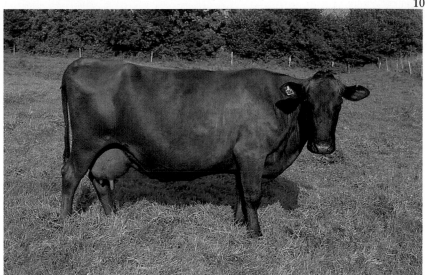

Angeln

Characteristics: Medium-framed. One colour, dark red to rich brown. Dark muzzle. Occasionally small white flecks on the udder. Dairy type upright, i.e. long and slim with light muscles. Naturally horned; most are de-horned.

	Bull	*Cow*
Height at shoulder	140–145	125–135
Weight	1100	550–630

Distribution: Angeln peninsula on the Baltic coast of Schleswig-Holstein. Has been crossed with many other breeds (Harz Red, Franconian, Glan, as well as cattle in the former Soviet Union, the Netherlands and other countries), which resulted in some cases in the original populations being almost displaced.

Uses: Dairy-based dual-purpose cattle. Good adaptability to extreme climates. Outstanding walking ability due to healthy constitution and good hooves. In 1983 the average milk production was 5280 kg (4.7% fat, 3.5% protein). Distinguished by particularly fine meat fibres. First calf produced at young age. Low rate of difficult calvings. Short period between calvings. High proportion of long-producing cows giving over 2000 kg milk fat.

Breed history: Arose in Angeln in the mid-nineteenth century from an old native land strain. In 1879 the Angeln cattle breeding association was founded. Production monitoring from 1902. The animals which weighed little more than 300 kg originally, became gradually much heavier. Since 1945 the Angeln and the other German red cattle strains have been combined under the 'Association of German Red Cattle Breeders'. The Angeln have sometimes been crossed with Red Danish cattle and blood from Sweden corresponding to the type.

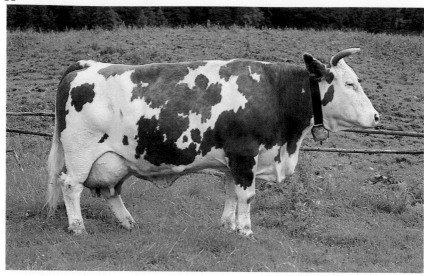

Spotted (Fleckvieh), Simmental

Characteristics: Medium to large cattle with strong bones and well-muscled. Spotted, occasionally with just a few white markings. The colour varies from pale gold to dark reddish brown. The head is always white in front of the eyes. The lower parts of the legs are also largely white. Horned.

	Bull	Cow
Height at shoulder	150–158	138–142
Weight	1200	750

Distribution: Alps and their foothills. South Germany. South-east Europe. Soviet Union. North and South America. UK. China. South Africa and other countries.

Uses: Dual-purpose breed with equal emphasis on milk and beef production.

The annual milk production of cows in herd book businesses in Germany is about 5100 kg (4.0% fat, 3.4% protein). Excellent fattening. The daily weight gain of fattening bulls on test stations is about 1300 g; about 63% carcase yield. Suited to all-purpose crossing with smaller breeds. In overseas countries kept mostly for beef.

Breed history: Goes back to animals in the Bernese Oberland, which were known as early as the Middle Ages as large, spotted cattle. From here, the 'Simmentals' spread into western and northern Switzerland. During the eighteenth century, and especially early in the nineteenth century, they came to Germany. Imported into Austria from 1830, where they are now the most numerous breed, accounting for 75% of the population.

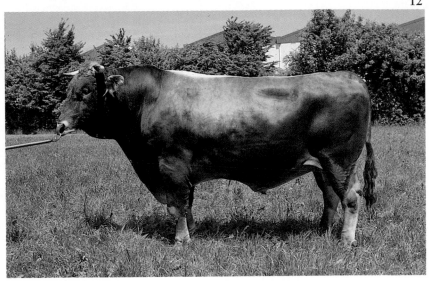

Brown Swiss

Characteristics: Medium-sized and medium-weight breed. Uniformly brown or grey-brown. The bulls are darker than the cows. Tips of horns, muzzle and hoofs have dark pigmentation. Eyes and muzzle pale-rimmed. Well-muscled with relatively fine bone formation. Horned.

	Bull	*Cow*
Height at shoulder	150–160	135–142
Weight	1000–1200	600–700

Distribution: Large areas of the Alps and their foothills. Now kept almost world-wide due to high milk yield and ease of adaptation to different climates and husbandry conditions. Main region of Germany where they are kept is the Allgäu.

Uses: Dairy-based dual-purpose cattle. Produces ten times its bodyweight in milk per year, i.e. 6000–7000 kg (4.0% fat, 3.7% protein). High return on investment. The daily weight gain of fattening bulls is about 1100–1200 g; 62% carcase yield. Early first calving age. Long-lived.

Breed history: Breeding started 600 years ago in central Switzerland. From there it spread into the eastern half of Switzerland and neighbouring areas (Württemberg, Allgäu, Vorarlberg and Tyrol, as well as the Italian Alps). The first dairy production tests were carried out in 1870. At this time, the first animals went to North America. While the Brown cattle in Germany became smaller, in North America larger animals with improved milk yields were bred. Since the mid-1960s, they have been used to improve the constitution and milking of the European Brown.

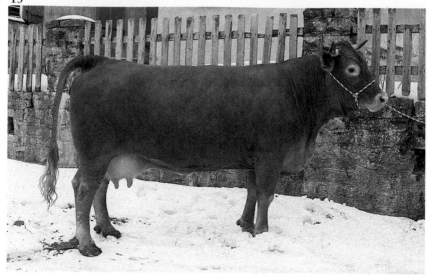

German Yellow, Franconian

Characteristics: Large cattle, well-muscled with strong bones. All light brown. Muzzle generally light, but sometimes dark. Horned.

	Bull	*Cow*
Height at shoulder	148–155	134–140
Weight	1150–1300	650–800

Distribution: Franconia (mainly Lower Franconia), the former East Germany (mainly Thüringer Wald), North and South America, South Africa.

Uses: Beef-based dual-purpose breed. Outside Germany kept primarily for beef. Puts on weight easily. Easy to feed. Easy calving. Long useful life. Annual milk production of herd book holdings 4700 kg (3.9% fat, 3.5% protein). Daily weight gain of fattening bulls is about 1200–1300 g, producing best quality meat and high carcase yield.

Breed history: At the beginning of the nineteenth century, Heilbronn cattle, a cross between red Land cattle and reddish brown Bern cattle, were introduced into Franconia. Around 1870 there was still a great variety of breeds there, golden brown strains being predominant. In 1872 a clear breeding aim was developed. The golden Franconian was developed by crossing with Simmentals, South Devons and Shorthorns. When the breed association was founded in 1897, it was decided there would be no more interbreeding. After World War II they were crossed with Red Danish and Red Flemish. There was always exchange with other golden cattle breeds (Limpurg, Glan-Donnersberg). Largely displaced the Austrian Golden cattle strains. The total population is falling rapidly as some individual populations are being either given up or converted to 'spotted' with Spotted cattle. Some inseminations with semen from Red Fleming cattle have been performed recently.

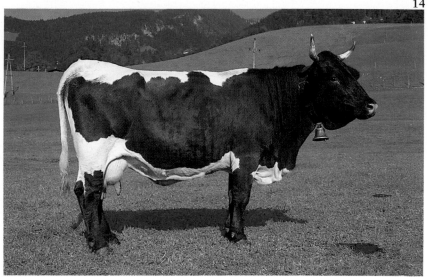

Pinzgau

Characteristics: Medium-sized with noticeably long body. Chestnut brown with broad white band beginning at the shoulder, running along the back and rear of the thighs and continuing along the belly and lower brisket. The tail is also white. Also white bands ('bandages') across the lower rear leg and usually across the top of the front leg. Muzzle and hooves dark. Short head. Good depth to brisket and flanks. Noticeable muscling of thigh. Horned.

	Bull	Cow
Height at		
shoulder	140–145	130–135
Weight	1000–1100	600–700

Distribution: Mainly Austria and Eastern Europe. In Bavaria, east and south of the Inn river.

Uses: Valued in the tropics and steppes as well as in extremely cold regions and in high Alpine zones. Easy to feed. Hardy. Placid. Good leg structure. Hard hooves. Outside German-speaking countries usually kept for beef. Suitable for all-purpose crossing. Dual-purpose cattle with equal emphasis on dairy and beef. Average annual milk yield is about 5000kg (3.8% fat, 3.5% protein). Good milker. Daily weight gain of fattening bull 1300 g. Top quality meat.

Breed history: Arose in the middle of the 19th century by cross-breeding of Valais cattle with native land races of Austria. This breed took its name from Pinzgau, a region of Salzburg. Originally triple-purpose cattle (meat, milk, work). In Austria, still the most frequent cattle breed in 1957. Numbers fell considerably there and in Germany after World War II. In recent years there has been cautious crossing with the Red Holstein. The world population of 1.3 million resides in a total of 25 states.

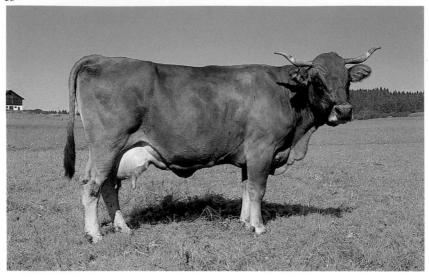

Murnau-Werdenfels

Characteristics: Uniformly straw coloured to dark golden; reddish brown is also possible. Pale back line. Dark muzzle, pale-rimmed. Darker animals have black 'masks'. Dark tail brush. Hooves and tips of horns black.

	Bull	Cow
Height at shoulder	138–145	128–130
Weight	850–950	500–600

Distribution: Murnauer Moos, Werdenfelser Land and the region of Mittenwald in Upper Bavaria.

Uses: Robust old land race. Undemanding. Lively. Hard hooves. Strong joints. Annual milk yield of about 4300 kg (3.8% fat, 3.4% protein), largely on farm's own fodder. Very prolific and long-lived.

Breed history: Presumably originates in the Tyrol and was introduced into its present range by Ettal and other monasteries. Examination of blood groups has revealed that it is closely related to the Brown. When breeding became aimed at high productivity in the mid-nineteenth century, the Murnau–Werdenfels was heavily displaced by the Brown and Spotted which lived close by to the west and east. There was a definite decline at the turn of the century, which nearly led to the collapse of the breed when tuberculosis and brucellosis were rife in the 1950s and 1960s. It was not recognised that harsh climatic conditions and poor feeding restrict the milk yield of this breed, so its considerable productivity only becomes evident in suitable situations. There are now just over 500 animals, of which 240 are cows. The breed is fostered by compensation for keeping the animals and premiums for covering and selective breeding.

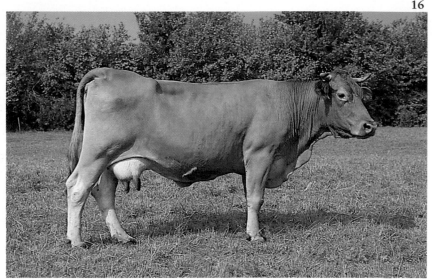

Limpurg

Characteristics: Medium-framed cattle with fine bone structure and moderate muscling. Relatively short, finely drawn head. Slender neck. Powerful shoulders The colour ranges from pale golden to reddish gold. The belly and pubic region as well as the insides of the thighs, around the eyes and inside the ears are lighter than the rest of the body. The muzzle is flesh coloured. Horns and hooves are golden.

	Bull	Cow
Height at		
shoulder	143	135
Weight	850–900	550–600

Distribution: Heuchlingen and region east of Stuttgart.
Uses: Fattens well. The meat has fine fibres, is tender and well-marbled. Hard, tough hooves. The milk yield of present day cows is just over 4000 kg.

Breed history: Its name comes from the place of origin, the county of Limpurg. Later it was kept in the region of Schwäbisch–Gmünd, Aalen and Gaildorf, mainly by the river Lein. At least since the beginning of the nineteenth century the Limpurgs have been described as all-golden cattle; at that time they were a small, dainty land race. Since the end of the century, large numbers of Golden Franconian and Glan–Donnersbergs were used. The Limpurgs are nevertheless noticeably smaller and daintier than Franconian cattle, presumably as a result of appropriate selection. The first societies for preserving and fostering Limpurg cattle were founded in 1890 in Aalen and Gaildorf, and in 1891 in Schwäbisch–Gmünd. The number of Limpurgs has been falling continuously since the start of the twentieth century. Before World War II there were 13,000 animals, and in 1952 there were only 5,000. Today there are few cattle of predominantly Limpurg stock.

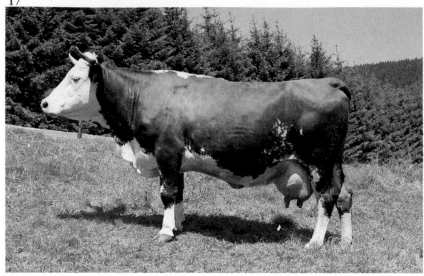

Vorderwälder

Characteristics: Small cattle with fine bone structure. Dark red and white. Sometimes without patches, but head and legs are still predominantly white. Resembles Spotted cattle in appearance, but not in frame. Horned.

	Bull	*Cow*
Height at		
shoulder	140	128–135
Weight	850–900	550–600

Distribution: Central and southern Black Forest, not on high land.

Uses: Suitable for grazing on meagre hill meadows. Can manage well on land that is poor in minerals. Calves easily. Long-lived. Lively. Dual-purpose breed with equal emphasis on milk and meat. Annual milk yield of HB cows is 4300 kg (4.0% fat, 3.4% protein). Daily weight gain of bulls at test stations is 1100 g. Fine, clear constitution with good articulation and excellent hooves permits grazing on steep slopes.

Breed history: The 'forest cattle' were first mentioned in 1829. Even then, a distinction was drawn between a large (today's Vorderwälder) and a smaller breed (today's Hinterwälder). In the mid-1960s it was decided to introduce the semen of four Ayrshire bulls. Milk and fat quantities were increased, at the slight expense of the fat content, but the muscling was poorer. As a specific blood line (B-line) soon asserted itself, it was decided to introduce six Red Holstein bulls. This cross-breeding gave an increase in milk quantity and content. There were also disadvantages, however, e.g. in constitution and poor hooves. Currently, Vorderwälders have an Ayrshire genetic content of 10%, and a Red Holstein genetic content of 15% (bulls) or 10% (heifers).

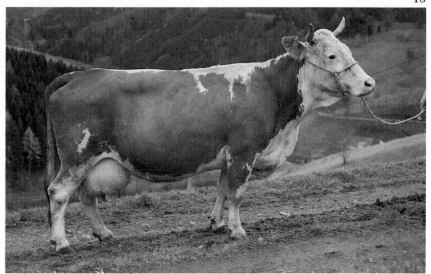

Hinterwälder

Characteristics: Fine, dainty cattle. Smallest cattle breed in central Europe. Golden to red. Mostly with patches, sometimes not. Head and legs are always white. Long middle hand. Clear, fine limbs. Horned.

	Bull	Cow
Height at shoulder	130	118–120
Weight	750	400–450

Distribution: The higher areas of the southern Black Forest (south of the Feldberg and around the Belchen). Some herds in Switzerland.

Uses: Suited to steep slopes, as they cause little erosion damage. Modest needs. Low susceptibility to illness. Long-lived. Calve easily. Suitable for keeping in Third World countries. The annual milk yield of herd book cows is 3100 kg (4.1% fat, 3.4% protein). On very good fodder, the yield may be 4000 kg or more. The daily weight gain of bulls kept for selective breeding was 805 g in 1980. High carcase yield. Top quality meat.

Breed history: Originally known on the right-bank Upper Rhine Plain as 'deer cattle', they were gradually displaced into the valleys of the southern High Black Forest. In 1888 the 'cattle breeding society for forest cattle' was founded. In 1914 this comprised about 1,000 members. For a long time they were scarcely influenced by other cattle breeds. Only in recent times has there been a cautious introduction of Vorderwälder blood, to meet the increased demand for a somewhat larger frame. The state of Baden–Württemberg pays owners husbandry premiums. A bank of deep-frozen semen has been established, both to create a gene reserve and to meet demand from outside the breed area. The total population is about 2,500 cows.

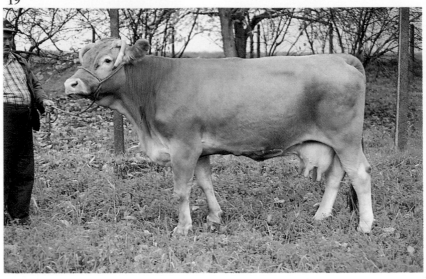

Glan

Characteristics: Medium-framed cattle. Uniformly pale golden to reddish brown. The area around the eyes and the muzzle as well as the underbelly and lower parts of the legs are lighter. Muzzle flesh-coloured. Horns and hooves golden to golden brown. Broad forehead. Horns slightly down-swept. Short nose. Broad, long pelvis. Powerful constitution.

	Bull	Cow
Height at shoulder	150	140
Weight	900–1000	600–700

Distribution: Rhineland–Palatinate in the region of the Glan river.

Uses: In the past they were good draught animals, well-suited to the soil and special climatic conditions. Easy to feed. Good growth. Long-lived. The annual milk yield is about 4000 kg (4.0% fat). Good meat quality. Very prolific.

Breed history: Arose in the 18th century from a small, single-colour land race by crossing with Charolais and Simmental. From the 1930s there was extensive exchange of blood with the neighbouring breeding areas, e.g. Lahn, and crossing with the Waldviertel Blond. After World War II there was interbreeding with the Franconian Golden. To improve milk yield, Red Danish and Angeln were used from 1950. The 'Association of Rhineland Glan cattle breeders' was disbanded in the mid-1960s. While the breed disappeared completely in the region of the Donnersberg, some Glan animals of the original type remained. In 1985 the 'Association for the preservation and fostering of Glan cattle' was founded. The state of Rhineland–Palatinate pays a breed preservation premium for each registered animal. After almost 20 years a Glan bull was bred selectively again in 1986.

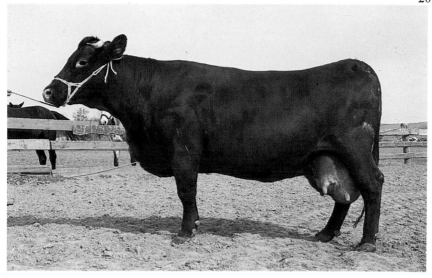

Harz Red

Characteristics: Medium-framed cattle. Reddish brown mono-colour, sometimes with white tail brush. Horns wax-yellow with dark tips.

	Bull	*Cow*
Height at shoulder	135–140	125–130
Weight	850–1000	550–600

Distribution: Western part of Harz.
Uses: Undemanding, robust, prolific and long-lived. Dual-purpose cattle with good muscling. The annual milk yield is on average 4500 kg (4.5% fat).
Breed history: In the sixteenth century many red Vogelsberg cattle were introduced into the Harz. At the end of the eighteenth century, 'Bernese cattle' (Simmental?) were brought in, and at the start of the nineteenth century, Zillertal cattle (possibly brown Tux cattle), which were distributed generally.

Then animals with white markings were excluded, and the present day type was produced. Emphasis was placed on performance as a draught animal. A herd book was set up for this breed at the turn of the century. The breeding aim was henceforth in conflict with the interests of the herdsmen, who wanted cattle that were not too large and which were capable of walking, so that they could be driven daily to the forest pasture. In 1942 the breed society of this breed joined with the Association of Angeln Cattle Breeders and those of other red cattle strains to form the 'Society of German Red Cattle Breeders'. Crossing with Red Danish cattle and later with Angeln cattle made the frame considerably larger and increased the milk yield and the fat content. There are few animals with the original blood stock left.

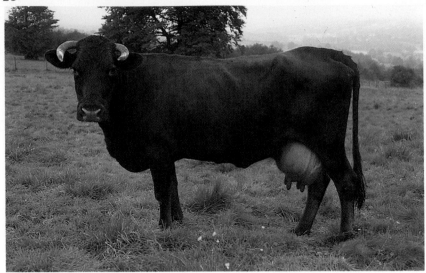

Volgelsberg

Characteristics: Medium-framed, well muscled. Mono-colour reddish brown hair. Pale muzzle. White tail switch surrounded by reddish brown hair. Light horns with dark tips.

	Bull	Cow
Height at shoulder	140	125–135
Weight	800–900	500–550

Distribution: Vogelsberg, occasionally in other parts of Hesse as well.
Uses: Placid. Robust. Long-lived. The average annual milk yield of 4000 kg (about 4.5% fat) is largely produced on the farm's own fodder. Good fattening capability and high-quality carcase. Still occasionally used as a draught animal.
Breed history: Stems from an old red German land race. Originally they were small-framed cattle, the cows weighing 400–450 kg, and their high milk yield was praised as early as the nineteenth century. Originally only occurring in the Vogelsberg, it eventually became popular in a wider locality. In 1885 a breed society for Vogelsberg cattle was founded. The breed was already often being displaced from the original breed area by Spotted cattle, and was sometimes crossed with them. After World War II it was crossed with Angeln. There are now only a few animals remaining which have predominantly Vogelsberg blood. The 'Association for the preservation and fostering of Red Hill cattle' is attempting to preserve it.

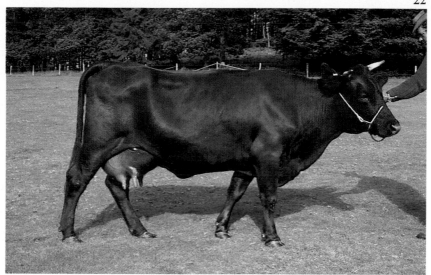

Wittgenstein

Characteristics: Medium-sized cattle. Reddish golden to reddish brown. White spots on the udder, belly and upper brisket (infrequent in modern animals). Horned.

	Bull	Cow
Height at shoulder	140	130
Weight	900–950	500–600

Distribution: Wittgenstein region (Westphalia), and neighbouring areas of Hesse.

Uses: Robust. Hardy. Dual-purpose cattle with equal emphasis on meat and milk. Annual milk yield about 4000 kg with a high fat content.

Breed history: Originally a native land race, mainly used as a draught breed. After World War II it was crossed with Angeln cattle. This improved the milk yield and the fat content.

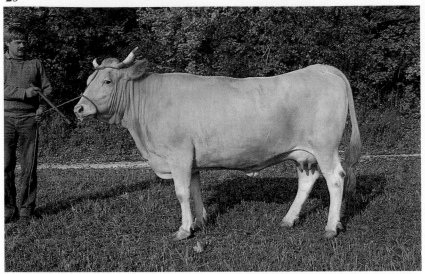

Blond Waldviertel

Characteristics: Medium-framed. Uniformly cream to flaxen, but also rust-coloured and white, with wax-coloured horns and hooves. Flesh-coloured muzzle. Crossing with other breeds has produced a predominantly light reddish brown. The horn tips are black. Long head. Small dewlap. Fine, short, soft, shiny hair.

	Bull	*Cow*
Height at shoulder	138	130
Weight	800–850	500–550

Distribution: Lower Austria.
Uses: Placid. Hardy. Tender meat.
Breed history: Can be traced back partly to Celtic cattle of the current area of distribution, and partly to central German Mountain cattle. In the nineteenth century there was inter-breeding with Scheinfeld (Franconian cattle) and Murboden cattle. Between 1938 and 1945 they were cross-bred with Glan–Donnersberg and Golden Franconian. From 1939 there was selective breeding and central sales events were held. After World War II there was again increased cross-breeding with Glan–Donnersberg, as they seemed to be a suitable size. Later, however, Golden Franconian bulls were again used, and altered the breed considerably. In 1954, 29% of the cattle in Lower Austria were of this breed. Displaced by the Spotted with its higher milk yield, the Blond Waldviertel was forced to outlying regions and the higher areas of the Waldviertel. The breed society was disbanded in 1966. A nuclear herd is kept to the south of Vienna.

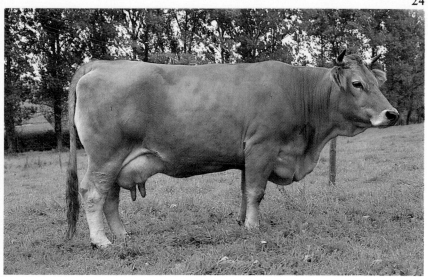

Murboden

Characteristics: Cows have a flaxen-coloured body that is sometimes reddish. The udder, the backs of the rear legs, the lower parts of the legs, and the area around the muzzle and the eyes are almost white. A pale triangle (flash) on the otherwise slate-blue muzzle is typical. Dark tail switch. Black hooves. Bulls are generally darker with a pale saddle spot. Horned: pale with dark tips.

	Bull	Cow
Height at shoulder	138–145	130–140
Weight	900–1000	550–650

Distribution: Styria. Carinthia. Lower Austria. Slovenia (Yugoslavia).
Uses: Good constitution from living in the Alps. Hardy. Good stamina. In the past they were excellent draught animals. Long-lived. Average annual milk yield of 4000 kg (4.2% fat). Good fatteners. The daily weight gain of fattening bulls is about 1300 g. Meat is of particularly good quality. Prolific.
Breed history: Arose in the valley basin of the River Mur from Mountain Spotted and the earlier Mürztal strain. Widely distributed in Austria in the past. Initially, the colour varied in accordance with the genetic content of constituent breeds: from grey through flaxen to fox red. After recognition as the fourth Styrian land race in 1869, selection was aimed at producing the present colour. The breeding target was established when the society was founded at the turn of the century. After that, there was no interbreeding with other breeds for a long time. After World War II it was considerably displaced by more productive breeds. The remaining population was heavily crossed with Franconian cattle. Today it is one of the Golden cattle. Recently some animals of the original type were taken into state keeping.

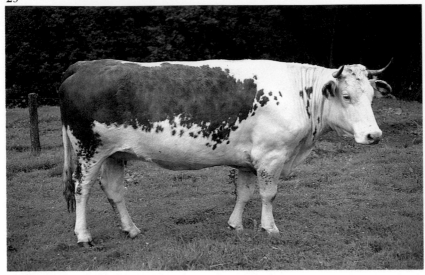

Ennstal Mountain Spotted

Characteristics: Light, dainty cattle. Predominantly white. Light red spots of pigmentation on thighs, flanks and side of breast. Spotted particularly at the transition to the non-pigmented areas. Ears mainly red. Horns and hooves golden. Small dewlap.

	Bull	Cow
Height at shoulder	140	130–135
Weight	800–850	450–550

Distribution: Styria.
Uses: Placid. Tough. Hardy. Good-quality meat.
Breed history: Derived from indigenous cattle that were originally mainly fox red. They are the descendants of the Bavarian cattle from the migratory era. Over time, more white markings appeared through selection, first only on the head and nape of the neck (helmets). Later, the whole neck and other parts of the body became white. The breed has been undergoing displacement by others since the eighteenth century. In 1880 it occurred in only a few valleys, so in 1895 giving up the breed completely was considered for the first time. The first Mountain Spotted society was founded in 1902. At about the turn of the century, however, they began to be displaced by crossing with Spotted cattle. From 1928 they belonged to the 'Mountain Spotted/Spotted cattle breed society'; pure Mountain Spotted were still included in the herd book. In 1935 there were pure-bred animals only in Ennstal. Scarcely any pure-bred bulls were used. After World War II, only one breeder kept Mountain Spotted. The last two pure-bred cows were slaughtered in October 1986. Mountain Spotted formed the basis for the Pinzgau cattle breed.

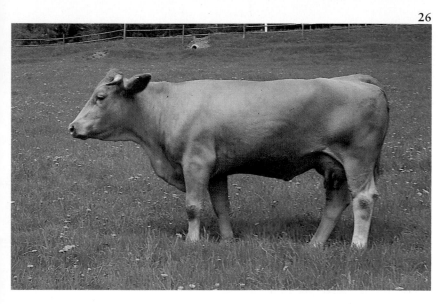

Carinthian Blond

Characteristics: Medium-sized, powerfully built. Uniform colouring, varying from white or silvery white to maize. No markings. Muzzle and eyelids are usually flesh pink, sometimes with blue to black pigmentation. Hooves and horns wax-coloured or have dark lines or tips.

	Bull	*Cow*
Height at shoulder	138–145	128–135
Weight	800–850	500–600

Distribution: Carinthia. Slovenia.
Uses: Fattens well. Outstanding meat quality. Robust health. Undemanding. Very prolific. Hard worker. Long-lived.
Breed history: Arose from mixing of pale and greyish golden cattle of hunno-slavic origin with Red and Red Spotted cattle of south German origin, which had predominated earlier in Carinthia. From the end of the 18th century it spread quickly in Carinthia and in parts of Styria. It represents the transition from the Hungarian steppe breeds to the mountain breeds. An important area of origin was the Lavant valley and the upper Gurk valley. Here, a breeding base was established on the Meierhofen estate near Freisach, which was to become very influential: the Marienhof strain. First there were some other strains (Maltlin strain, Katschtal strain etc.). At the start of the 20th century there was crossbreeding with the golden Franconian and the Spotted. In 1930 the Blond cattle population constituted 37% of the cattle population in Carinthia. In 1938 the previously independent breed societies combined to form the 'Südmark Blond cattle society'. After World War II there was isolated crossbreeding with Red Friesians, and later with Golden Franconian cattle. Finally it was virtually displaced by other breeds.

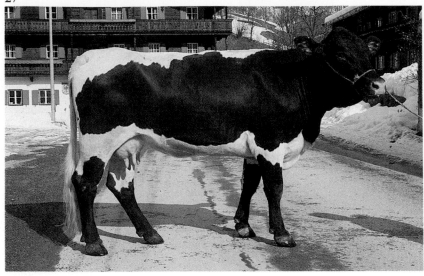

Jochberg Hummeln

Characteristics: Medium-sized. Chestnut brown. A white band begins at the withers and runs over the rump, the hindquarters and the belly to the dewlap. The tail and the udder are also white. Usually, white bands across the tops of the legs ('bandages'). Relatively long head. Narrow forehead, almost pointed in the middle. Dark hooves. Powerfully built. Deep brisket. Well-muscled. Polled.

	Bull	Cow
Height at shoulder	150	135–148
Weight	900–1000	600–650

Distribution: Only found in one agricultural operation near Kitzbühel in Austria.

Uses: Good-natured. Sure-footed. High carcase yield. Top-quality meat. Respectable milk yield from basic fodder; average annual milk yield about 4300 kg (4.0% fat).

Breed history: Derived from Pinzgau cattle. The first documented hornless animal was born in 1834, in the area where these cattle now live. In the 1840s these cattle were fashionable for a time in Kitzbühel and were also in demand for export. At the end of the last century, only a few owners remained, and by 1929 there was only one, who had in fact always bred the 'Hummeln'. The animals are still kept here. The owner alternates bought-in horned Pinzgaus and hornless bulls of his own. Some years ago the population had fallen to 2 cows; now there are about 15 animals. Only once in recent decades has an animal been sold, except for slaughter. Hornless animals of originally horned species are called 'Hummeln' in the Brixen valley in Tyrol; this applies to sheep and goats as well as cattle.

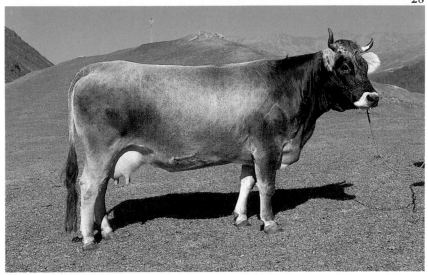

Tyrolean Grey

Characteristics: Silver to steel-grey, sometimes with a hint of brown. Darker shading around the eyes, on the neck and shoulders and on the outsides of the thighs. The area around the muzzle, the underside of the body, the udder and the insides of the legs are lighter. Bulls are darker and often have white saddles. Dark hooves and horns.

	Bull	Cow
Height at shoulder	133	120–125
Weight	900–1000	500–550

Distribution: North and South Tyrol. Occasionally in Allgäu. Recently a few animals in Switzerland.
Uses: Robust. Placid. Hard hooves. Dual-purpose breed. Average annual milk yield is 3800 kg (4.0% fat); the peak yield is about 7000 kg. The yield is remarkable in that 85% of all Grey breeding farms are above 1000 m and most of the Alpine pastures are at 1600–2000 m. Average daily weight gain of fattening animals is 1150 g. High carcase yield of over 60%. Good fodder utilisation. Matures early. Calves without complications.
Breed history: Ancient indigenous breed. In Roman times the Ligurian–Rhaetian Grey from the upper Inn valley was known for its high milk yield. The breed range extended over large parts of the eastern Alps 100 years ago. The 'Upper Inn valley Grey cattle breed society' was founded at the start of this century. Tyrolean Grey made a large contribution to the improvement of cattle breeds in south-eastern Europe and Italy. The first Grey cattle breed association was founded in 1922. Decreasing number of animals as the Tyrolean Grey is increasingly displaced into sparse regions in side valleys of the original area of distribution.

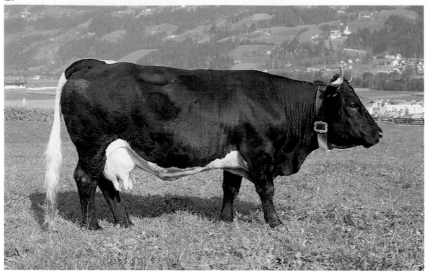

Tux

Characteristics: Black or rich reddish brown (Zillertal type) with white markings on pelvis and base of tail, milk escutcheon and on the udder and underbelly. The end of the tail is also white. Occasionally there are white bands across the tops of the legs. Area around the muzzle is pale. Short, broad head with thick horns. Short legs. Broad, compact well-muscled torso.

	Bull	Cow
Height at shoulder	140	120–130
Weight	800–900	550–600

Distribution: Ziller valley (Tyrol).
Uses: Undemanding. Strong desire to fight, which used to lead to fighting among the cows when they were first released onto the high summer pasture (cow play-off). The winner became the leader of the herd for the duration of the summer on the high pasture. Good fattener.

Breed history: Thought to be descended from the Eringer. Originally it was kept in large areas of Tyrol, but in the nineteenth century it became restricted to the Ziller valley. In the past it was selected for its desire to fight. This unusual breeding target caused milk yield to be neglected. The collapse of the breed began with the systematic campaign against tuberculosis. The reduction of numbers associated with the destruction of positive reactants could not be overcome by the breed. There are now only remnants of the breed remaining. Tux cattle were involved in the creation of the Russian breeds Gorbatov, Red Tambov and Yurinov. Recently a society was founded in the Ziller valley for fostering Tux cattle.

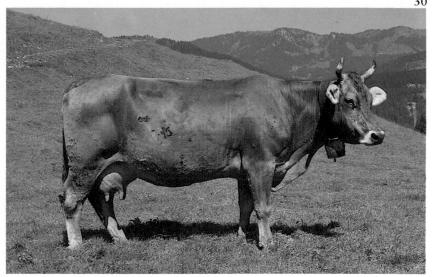

Montafon, Vorarlberg Brown
old breed

Characteristics: Medium-weight. Heavy build. Deep torso. Strong bone structure. Well muscled. Deep, broad pelvis. Base of tail slightly raised. Mostly medium to dark brown. Pale back line. Almost white around the muzzle. Hair inside ears is pale. Muzzle, hooves and horn tips are dark. Nicely curved, medium-length horns.

	Bull	*Cow*
Height at shoulder	136	128
Weight	750–1000	500 600

Distribution: Vorarlberg. Similar forms in Tyrol and Allgäu.

Uses: Average annual yield of herd book cows in 1982 was 5092 kg milk (3.9% fat). The old breed is not recorded separately. It is to be assumed that they do not quite achieve the milk yield quoted. Long-lived. Robust. Accustomed to living in the mountains. Low susceptibility to udder diseases.

Breed history: Original breeding area in southern Vorarlberg (Montafon valley) and neighbouring regions. In the second half of the nineteenth century adopted largely in the pure form in large areas of Vorarlberg. Then crossed with other Brown strains. Aroused interest at the world exhibition in Vienna in 1873. The very dark colour of some of the present day Brown animals may be due to Montafon blood. Now only about 200 mainly old animals not crossed with Brown Swiss. Abroad, the Vorarlberg Brown is often considered to be a Montafon up to the time when it was crossed with the Brown Swiss. At this point, the animals – irrespective of whether they are really Montafon or just Brown – can be cited as an example of a remnant of an original type uninfluenced by American blood.

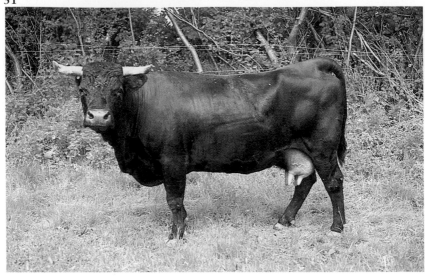

Eringer

Characteristics: Strong constitution. The hair is dark red to black/brown. Spotted animals are rare. Short, broad head with concave forehead line. Fine limbs. Well muscled. Powerful horns.

	Bull	*Cow*
Height at shoulder	125–134	118–128
Weight	650–750	480–530

Distribution: Canton of Valais in Switzerland.

Uses: Undemanding. Adaptable. Suitable for mountain areas. Notable for its readiness to fight, which is often the reason for keeping it. Cows and heifers are placed in five weight classes and allowed to fight in spring. The winner in all classes in the final fights brings high regard to her owner; such animals command a high price. Bulls are often used for all-purpose crossing or for initial serving of heifers of other breeds. Beef-based dual-purpose breed. The annual milk yield is 3100 kg (3.7% fat), considerable when one takes into account the special husbandry conditions and fodder available.

Breed history: It is thought to have come to the region of modern Valais with the Romans. In 1884 a homogeneous breeding standard was created. In 1917 the Association of the Eringer breed cooperative was founded. Over the centuries, Eringer cattle have provided the basis for several other breeds in the Alpine region. The population has declined gradually in the past 40 years. A majority of the breed is kept as secondary business.

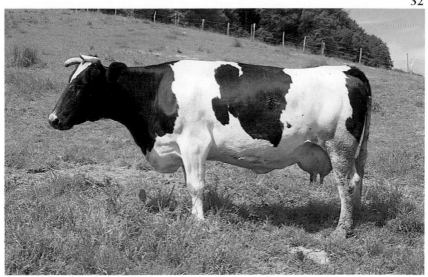

Black and White

Characteristics: Medium-framed. White with black patches. Head black with white markings. Legs mainly white. Medium-muscled. Horned.

	Bull	Cow
Height at shoulder	154–160	140–145
Weight	1000–1200	650–750

Distribution: Canton of Freiburg and neighbouring regions in western Switzerland.

Uses: Dairy-based dual-purpose cattle. The average annual milk yield is 5700 kg (3.8% fat). The cows generally produce their first calf at 28 months. The birth weight of calves is on average 43.3 kg.

Breed history: Up to the middle of the nineteenth century, black/brown and red/brown cattle were kept together in the same enterprise in Switzerland. Only after 1870 were the two colour groups separated. At the same time, the first breed cooperative of the Black and White was founded. Owing to increased demand for Simmentals, abroad as well as at home, the originally extensive breeding range of the Black and White shrank to the Greyerzerland and the neighbouring regions of the canton of Freiburg. Up to the start of the 1960s they were largely genetically independent of all other Friesian populations. Then they were crossed with European Friesians. From 1966 there was large-scale use of semen from the Holstein–Friesian breed in North America. This largely displaced the original breed. The genetic content of Freiburg Black and White in the Friesians currently kept in the breeding region is estimated to be 15%.

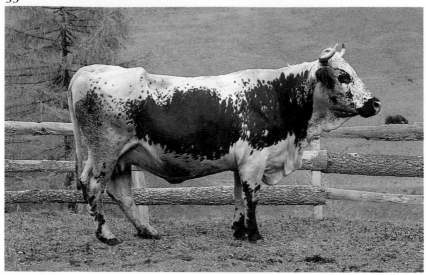

Pustertal Spotted

Characteristics: Predominantly white. On the sides of the body, especially the flanks, there are black, chestnut brown or light brown areas, which break up at the transition to the white skin, so in many animals there are numerous small pigmented spots of skin here. These parts look as though they have been sprayed with colour. This gives rise to the name 'sprayed' for animals thus marked. Depending on the colour and the part of the body affected by the pigmentation, they used to be called black- or red-sprayed, and head– or body-sprayed. Horned.

	Bull	Cow
Height at shoulder	135–145	125–135
Weight	800–900	500–600

Distribution: Puster valley and its side valleys, South Tyrol. Recently there have been a few examples in Germany.

Uses: The average annual milk yield is about 3000 kg. It has to be taken into account that the animals are kept in harsh conditions and live on sparse home-produced fodder.

Breed history: Arose from the crossing of Eringer cattle with the indigenous red land race in the Puster valley. At one time they were distributed over the whole of Pustertal. In the 19th century they were crossed with Pinzgaus. The demise of the breed started when in 1927 a decree from the agricultural inspectorate excluded them from selective breeding. There are only about 80 cows, kept on 15 farms. Some years ago, several animals were taken to Germany and distributed among several populations. The breed is flourishing there. Furthermore, semen samples and embryos have been stored.

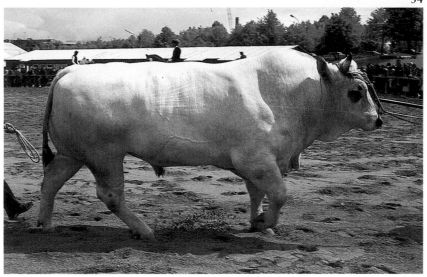

Chianina

Characteristics: Largest breed of cattle in the world. A homogeneous porcelain-white, occasionally with a hint of grey. Eyelashes and tail brush are black. Skin is pigmented, so areas with little hair (eyelids, anus, vulva) are dark. Muzzle, hooves and horns also dark. Very long body. Narrow, fairly long head. Short, smooth hair. Calves are born reddish golden, and do not change colour until 2 months old. There are four strains, differing in size and weight.

	Bull	*Cow*
Height at shoulder	160–180	150–170
Weight	1200–1500	800–1000

Distribution: In Italy mainly in the area between Florence and Rome and between Pisa and Perugia. North America. In Germany they are not kept as a pure breed; bulls are used for cross-breeding programmes.

Uses: In the past they were powerful draught animals, and are occasionally used as such today. They are kept as a beef breed in suckler cow herds. High carcase yield. Good-quality meat. Little tendency to put on fat. Heat-tolerant. Not disease-prone.

Breed history: The oldest cattle breed in Italy. The world record for live-weight cattle was set in 1955 in Arezzo by the bull 'Donetto' at 1740 kg. The resemblance to cattle in Etruscan drawings is noticeable, so there is thought to be a genealogical connection. They originally came from Umbria in Upper Italy, but the current type was developed in the Chianina valley in Tuscany. An official breeding programme commenced in 1932 with state support. Performance attributes were just as important as the white colour for inclusion in the herd book. Their importance as working animals is declining in Italy. There is now emphasis on beef production.

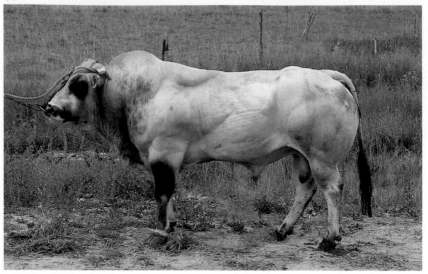

Piemontese

Characteristics: Medium-sized. Cows are light grey with a dark muzzle and anus and dark vulva. Bulls are darker overall, especially the withers, the upper part of the front legs, around the eyes and the tail brush. Powerful muscles at the nape of the neck, withers and haunches. Relatively fine-boned. Horned. Calves are born reddish-golden and change colour when they are a few months old.

	Bull	Cow
Height at shoulder	140	130
Weight	800	500–600

Distribution: Mainly western Upper Italy. There is an export ban on breeding cattle; outside Italy, only semen of Piemontese bulls is obtainable.
Uses: Pure beef breed, often having double muscling on the loins. High daily weight gain. The carcase yield is up to 65%. Good carcase quality. Very little fat.
Breed history: The only European breed to have zebu blood. In 1848 in the region of Piedmont, several cattle strains were united in the 'Razza Piemontese': the large, golden cattle of the plain with long legs, and the small, red to straw-coloured Demont strain kept in the mountains. The first were draught and beef cattle, but gave only a modest amount of milk. In addition there were the Albese, which already produced double-loined calves, as well as another strain. Originally a triple-purpose breed, but the working ability lost its importance first. During the past 25 years the dairy aspect has also declined, resulting in the modern type.

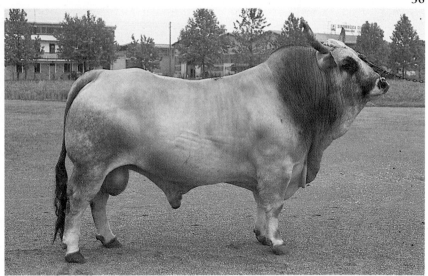

Romagnola

Characteristics: Large-framed cattle. The cows are white to light grey, while the bulls have more intense colouring; the neck and the area around the eyes are particularly dark. In both sexes the eyelids, anus, tail brush and muzzle are black, as is the vulva in female animals. Calves are reddish-golden in their first months of life. Heavily muscled. Horned.

	Bull	*Cow*
Height at shoulder	155	145
Weight	1100–1200	650–750

Distribution: Italy, especially the Apennines and lower Po plain.
Uses: Adaptable. Undemanding. Originally triple-purpose cattle with strong emphasis on draught aspect. Today it is bred purely for beef. The daily weight gain of fattening animals is about 1300 g. Top-quality carcase. Little tendency to put on fat. Scarcely any calving difficulties.

Breed history: Arose from the crossing of Podolic cattle with indigenous strains. They were consolidated in the nineteenth century in the province of Forlì. They were crossed with Chianina during the period 1850–80. At the world exhibition in Paris in 1900 the Romagnola was distinguished as the best fattening breed. A herd book was opened in 1956. There are two types of the breed: the 'Romagnola gentile' strain kept on the plain grows faster and matures earlier, the 'Romagnola di Montagna' strain kept in the mountains is the better working animal.

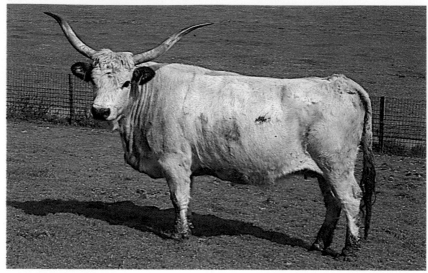

Hungarian Steppe

Characteristics: Large-framed. Silver white to ash grey. Often darker colouring around eyes, withers, sides of belly and haunches, especially in bulls. Calves are born reddish golden. Narrow and relatively short head. Long, flat neck. Pronounced withers. Back often sags slightly. Long, deep brisket. Sloping pelvis. Relatively small udder. Remarkably long, wide-spreading horns, up to 80 cm long in bulls.

	Bull	Cow
Height at shoulder	150	135–145
Weight	900	500–650

Distribution: Hungary. Small numbers in other central and East European countries.
Uses: Outstanding draught animal. Matures late. Calves easily. Resistant to disease. Long-lived. Undemanding. Very hard hooves. Calves grow quickly. Annual milk yield is about 2000 kg. Recently females often used for the production of fattening cattle.
Breed history: Diverging views on their origins. It is assumed that either the Magyars brought these cattle with them from eastern Europe in the ninth century, or they came later from the east or the south (Balkans, Italy). From the fourteenth to the eighteenth century these cattle were a valued beef breed way beyond Hungary. They were particularly popular in Italy, Austria and Germany, mainly in the markets of Venice, Nuremberg, Augsburg and Vienna. When agriculture was intensified in the nineteenth century, the Steppe became an outstanding draught animal. The population has fallen since the end of the nineteenth century. It reached a low point of 187 cows and 6 bulls. In Hungary there are now 1,000 animals.

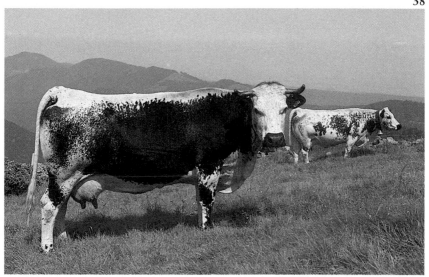

Vosges

Characteristics: The basic colour is black. There is a white dorsal stripe (finching), a white tail and white underside, and the legs are white from the carpal and tarsal joints down. The edges of the pigmented area are either sharply defined or flecked. The head is mainly milky grey. Dark rings around the eyes. The muzzle and the area around it are also dark.

	Bull	Cow
Height at shoulder	135–140	125–136
Weight	900–1000	550–600

Distribution: Vosges, France.
Uses: Good-natured. Robust. Undemanding (mountain cattle). Fed almost exclusively on home-grown fodder. In the summer they are kept on high land in the Vosges. Milk-based dual-purpose cattle; 600 cows subject to milk monitoring (in all there are 7000 cows). Annual milk yield on average 3300 kg (3.8% fat).

Breed history: As the original breed in this form since at least the start of the nineteenth century in the Vosges. After the Thirty Years War, Swedish soldiers brought Jemtländer, a Swedish breed similar to the Vosges in colouring, into the region. At the end of the nineteenth century they were crossed with cattle from Lothringen, which were similar to the Vosges cattle but heavier. In the past there were also brown animals, but they could not be used for breeding as a result of an official order. In 1974 semen from Telemark bulls in Norway was first used to a very limited extent.

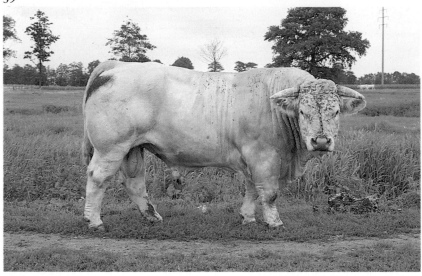

Charolais

Characteristics: Medium- to large-framed beef cattle. The body is very deep and broad. The colour is white to cream, the muzzle being pink and the hooves pale. Short, broad head. Heavily muscled loins and haunches. Horned.

	Bull	Cow
Height at shoulder	142–155	135–140
Weight	1100–1400	700–900

Distribution: France and most other European countries, especially UK, North and South America, and many other countries across the world (about 60 in all).

Uses: Put on weight fast. Little tendency to put on fat. Good-quality meat. High carcase yield. Excellent meat conformation, especially of the valuable parts. On fattening test stations, average weight gains of 1300–1600 g per day are achieved. Mature for slaughter relatively late, therefore well suited to fattening for high finished weight. Good fodder utilisation. Mature late. Cows' first calvings can be difficult. Kept in herds of suckler cows. Well suited to all-purpose cross-breeding.

Breed history: Originated in a land race distributed around Charolles (France), and crossed with white Shorthorns in the nineteenth century. In 1864 a herd book was established by Conte de Bouillé in Nevers for the Nevers–Charolaise breed. Another herd book was started in 1882 in Charolles. They were combined in 1919 as the Charolais herd book. The breed attained international importance after World War II. The first animals arrived in Germany in about 1960. There is no cohesive breeding region there, but most of the animals are in the northern half of the country.

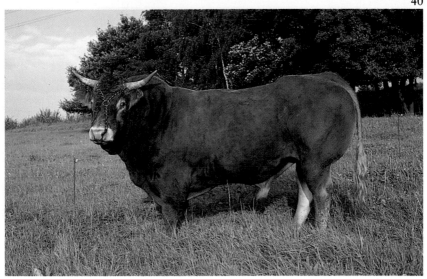

Limousin

Characteristics: Medium- to large-framed beef cattle of rectangular shape. The hair is all golden (straw-coloured) to reddish gold with lighter areas around the eyes and the muzzle as well as on the lower brisket. Bulls darker. Pink muzzle. Relatively small head. All meat-bearing parts of the body are heavily muscled. Pale horns and hooves.

	Bull	*Cow*
Height at shoulder	145–155	135–140
Weight	1000–1200	650–800

Distribution: Original breeding area in the middle of France (centred on the town of Limoges). Has been exported to many countries, Germany, mainly in the north and west.
Uses: Resistant to effects of the weather. Prolific. Long-lived. The annual milk yield is about 4100kg (4.0% fat, 3.2% protein). The Limousin is however kept in France mainly and in other countries exclusively for beef and is not milked; the cows rear their calves. The birth weight of male calves is on average 39kg and of female calves 36kg. Fattening animals show high daily weight gain (on average 1250 g). High carcase yield. Little tendency to put on fat. Meat is tender and fine-fibred. Few difficult births. Well suited to all-purpose cross-breeding.

Breed history: The organised breeding of the Limousin dates back to the 1860s. At that time its working attributes were predominant. A herd book was established in 1886. Conversion of the breed to beef cattle took place from 1900.

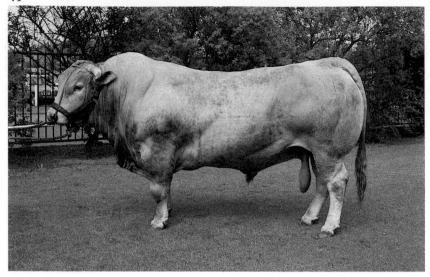

Blonde d'Aquitaine

Characteristics: Large-framed. Very long. Relatively small head. All pale golden to straw-coloured. Lighter areas around eyes and muzzle. Underside of body and lower parts of legs are lighter. The muzzle and the mucous membranes are pink. Very well developed muscles in all meat-bearing parts. Horns wax yellow with dark tips.

	Bull	Cow
Height at		
shoulder	150–152	140–145
Weight	1000–1250	700–850

Distribution: In the country of origin, France, mainly in the south-west. Kept in the most important meat-producing countries of the world, especially the USA, Argentina, Brazil and Australia. Individual animals can be found in Austria. At some insemination centres in south Germany there are individual bulls, whose semen is used with Brown cows to produce all-purpose calves.

Uses: Undemanding and robust. Adaptable. Long-lived. Neither sensitive to extreme temperatures nor to high precipitation. Length of the calves causes a few difficult births. Fast-growing. Good meat production capacity. Daily weight gains at the age of 6–12 months are 1400–1500 g. Although they mature early, little fat is laid down.

Breed history: Arose in 1962 when the three Blond breeds, Garounais, Quercy and Blonde des Pyrénées were united. These initial breeds were originally kept as draught animals, but were later bred for beef, in particular for veal production. In France there are breeding programmes using selective mating to improve meat quality and characteristics as mothers on the one hand, and to select bulls for crossing with dairy and land races on the other.

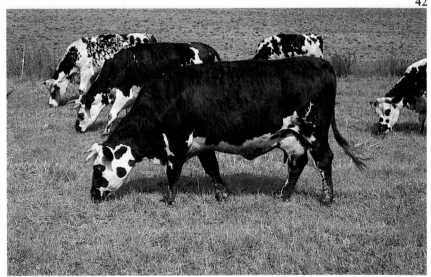

Normandy

Characteristics: Large-framed, very deep and broad. Well-muscled. Mostly distinctively marked, sometimes fully coloured. The triple colouring is notable. The basic shade of the pigmentation is mid-brown, often dark brown to almost black streaks or flecks. The head is mainly white. The eyes are often dark-rimmed, the pigmented muzzle likewise. The relatively short head has an indentation between the forehead and nose region, typical of the breed (*coup de poing*). Horned.

	Bull	Cow
Height at shoulder	150–160	135–145
Weight	1000–1300	600–800

Distribution: France, mainly Normandy and Brittany. Southwards to the Loire area. Isolated populations in other parts of France.

Uses: Dairy-based dual-purpose cattle. The annual milk yield is on average 4100 kg (4.2% fat, 3.6% protein). The daily weight gain of fattening bulls is on average 1300 g. The breed is suitable for the keeping of wet-nurse cows, the milk of a single cow being sufficient to rear three calves.

Breed history: It is assumed that the breed was brought to northern France by the Vikings in the ninth and tenth centuries. About 1850 it was crossed with the Shorthorn and expanded southwards by displacement cross-breeding. A herd book was established as early as 1883, which was followed by the first monitoring society in France in 1907. In 1920 the herd book was reorganised, and in 1946 it was decided to include all cows in the milk production study. To consolidate the breed further, the herd book for bulls was closed. In 1958 this breed accounted for one-quarter of the total cattle population of France. The percentage is now falling, however.

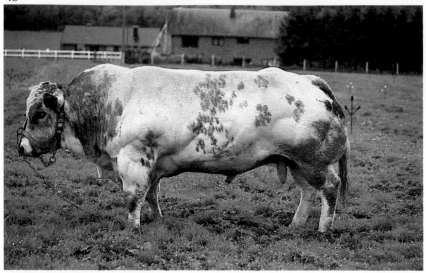

Belgian Blue and White

Characteristics: Medium-sized, heavy cattle, sometimes with massive musculature. The colours are blue, white, and blue and white. Sometimes there are black and white animals. Relatively small head. There is a dual-purpose type (beef/dairy) and a beef type.

	Bull	*Cow*
Height at shoulder	145–150	133–138
Weight	1100–1200	700–800

Distribution: Belgium. For a time they were kept in Germany as well, but the small number of breeders gave up keeping them because the calving difficulties had been underestimated.

Uses: The annual milk yield of the dual-purpose type is approximately 4000 kg (3.8% fat, 3.3% protein). Daily weight gains are about 1300 g. The carcase yield of the beef type is 65%, and of the dual-purpose type 60%. Top-quality carcase, especially in the double-loined ones. High proportion of valuable cuts. The proportion of difficult births is particularly high among cows calving for the first time. The necessary caesarian sections are often performed by the owner.

Breed history: Can be traced back to two different types of land strain. In the second half of the last century they were crossed with Charolais and Shorthorn. At first only a dual-purpose breed was sought. From 1950 some of the population was bred mainly for heavy muscling. Bulls are used for crossing with cows of dual-purpose breeds.

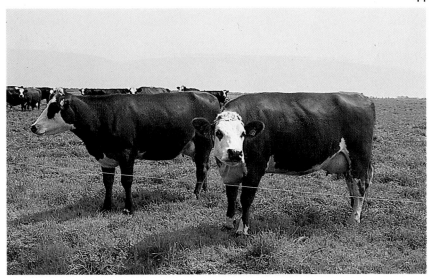

Groningen, Blaarkop

Characteristics: Medium-sized cattle with considerable depth and breadth of body. The majority of animals are black (about 60%), the rest are red. The head, lower brisket, udder and extremities are white. The eyes usually have dark areas around them (spectacles). The muzzle is dark. Horned.

	Bull	Cow
Height at shoulder	140–145	130–140
Weight	800–900	600–650

Distribution: Netherlands, mainly in the provinces of Groningen (the place of origin), South Holland, Utrecht and Gelderland. Exported to some other countries to improve the local cattle.

Uses: Dual-purpose cattle with good muscling and an average annual milk yield of approximately 6000 kg (4.1% fat, 3.5% protein). The best animals produce more than 100,000 kg of milk during their lives. The daily weight gain of fattening bulls is on average 1150 g. Very hard hooves.

Breed history: Arose from the old indigenous Friesian strain by crossing with Shorthorns in the second half of the last century. There were cattle with the typical colour distribution of this breed in the Netherlands in the fifteenth century. Originally more a beef animal, gradually developed into a dairy-based dual-purpose breed. The breed was officially recognised in 1906. Groninger now make up less than 1% of the cattle population of the Netherlands. The main reason is the crossing of Holstein Friesian or Red Holstein with the more common cattle populations of the Netherlands, which puts the Groningen at a disadvantage with regard to milk yield. In 1976 the 'Blaarkop working group' devised a plan to preserve the breed.

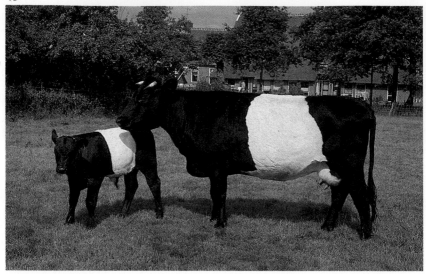

Lakenfelder (Dutch Belted)

Characteristics: Medium-framed. Head, neck, fore- and hind-quarters black (75% of animals) or brown (25%) without markings. A wide, white band runs around the middle of the body. Horned.

	Bull	Cow
Height at shoulder	135–140	125–135
Weight	900–1000	550–650

Distribution: Netherlands. Belgium. USA.

Uses: Dual-purpose cattle with an average annual milk yield of 5000 kg. Calves fatten well.

Breed history: Cattle with this characteristic colour pattern appear in paintings by Dutch masters of the seventeenth century. The first descriptions of animals with such markings date from the eighteenth century. When animals with the Lakenveld colouring appeared repeatedly in other cattle breeds, breeding stocks started to be built up systematically from the beginning of this century. A herd book was established in the Netherlands in 1918. They have been bred in the USA since 1850. After World War II, the number of animals declined sharply until some interested breeders made intensive efforts to preserve the breed. In the 1960s, a Belted Galloway bull was crossed, which, as expected, passed on the hornless characteristic of the breed. The breed experienced a great upsurge when the 'Stichting zeldzame huisdierrassen' was founded in 1976 and paid special attention to the cause of the Lakenvelder. There are now quite a number of breeders, although the number of well-marked animals is still limited.

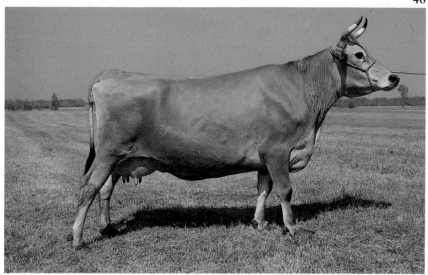

Jersey

Characteristics: Small, dainty cattle with fine bone structure and light muscling. The colour varies greatly: there are golden-brown to light red ones, as well as cream and almost black animals; occasionally some with patches. The head, shoulders and hips are almost always somewhat darker. There is often a back line. The dark muzzle almost always has a light ring around it. Short head with broad forehead. Concave forehead line. Large, expressive eyes. Horned. Generally the horn base of calves is destroyed, so that the animals remain hornless.

	Bull	Cow
Height at shoulder	127	120–125
Weight	700	350–400

Distribution: Almost world-wide. In Germany there is no cohesive breeding zone, but most are in the eastern half of Lower Saxony. Some Jerseys are kept in other cattle herds to increase the fat content of the milk output.

Uses: Single-purpose dairy breed. Herd book cows in Germany produced on average 4008 kg of milk in 1983 (6.0% fat, 4.2% protein). Milk yield is maintained well. Mature early. Calve easily. Long-lived.

Breed history: Originated on the Channel Island of Jersey. This breed has been known for the high fat content of its milk since the eighteenth century. It has not been crossed with other breeds since then. The first herd book society was established in 1866. Milk yield recording was introduced on the island of Jersey in 1912. Exports of animals to the USA began at the start of the nineteenth century, and later to England, New Zealand and Denmark. German Jersey rearing is based largely on imports from Denmark.

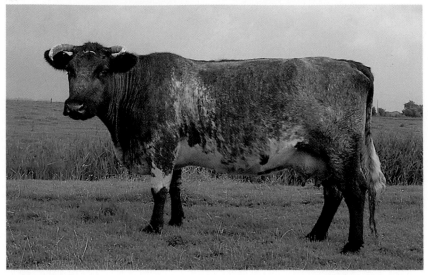

Shorthorn

Characteristics: Two types: dairy Shorthorn and beef Shorthorn. The body of the beef Shorthorn has the rectangular shape of all beef cattle breeds. Three colours: red, white and milky red. Animals with coloured hair have white flecks, especially on the underbelly. The horns stay quite short and are wax-coloured.

	Bull	*Cow*
Height at shoulder	140	130
Weight	700–900	500–600

Distribution: Originally the north-east of England (County Durham, among others). Now North and South America and many other countries.

Uses: The dairy Shorthorn is a dual-purpose animal, with an annual milk yield of on average 4800 kg (3.6% fat, 3.3% protein). The beef Shorthorn is kept in herds of suckler cows.

Breed history: The original area was known in the sixteenth century for large draught cattle with heavy muscling. In the eighteenth century, the **Colling** brothers bred the Shorthorns on the basis of several herds of large cattle with good milk yields. The first cattle herd book in the world (1822), and the first breed to be distributed world-wide. At the start of the nineteenth century the first animals arrived in North Germany. Somewhat later they were crossed with many cattle breeds of continental Europe. As there was no clear breeding target, bulls of the dairy and beef Shorthorn were used in the same herds. The consistency of the breed was therefore lost. Lost ground in UK and also in Germany, especially after World War II. On Eiderstedt there are only remnants in the hands of three breeders.

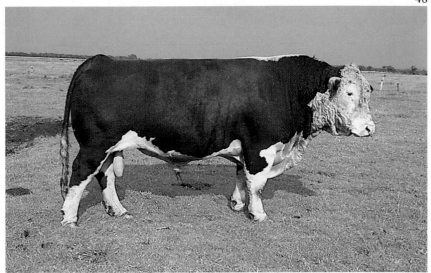

Hereford

Characteristics: Medium-framed cattle. The basic colour is red. The head and front of the neck, the brisket, underbelly, udder or scrotum, tail brush and lower parts of the legs, as well as a narrow stripe on the upper side of the neck to the withers, are white. Well-developed fore-quarters. Deep brisket. Relatively short legs. Most animals have horns (the horns typically curve down at the sides of the head), but there is a polled strain in North America and UK (Polled Hereford).

	Bull	*Cow*
Height at shoulder	130–140	125–135
Weight	800–900	500–600

Distribution: With over 5 million herd book animals in 56 countries, it is the most widely distributed beef cattle breed in the world. Primarily UK, North and South America, Australia, New Zealand, South Africa, but also many other countries.

Uses: Undemanding. Adaptable. Tolerant of climatic conditions. Daily weight gains of fattening bulls are on average 1100 g. Meat is not too fatty. Mature early. Calve easily.

Breed history: Ancient breed, kept in western England for centuries. It gained its modern appearance around 1800 by crossing with cattle from Flanders. Originally, Herefords were large-framed draught cattle. During the nineteenth century there was selective breeding for early maturity, which entailed a reduction in the size of the frame. The first herd book was published in 1846, and later adopted by the 'Hereford Herd Book Society', founded in 1878. The breed is still centred on the Hereford area. The first polled Herefords appeared in UK in 1955.

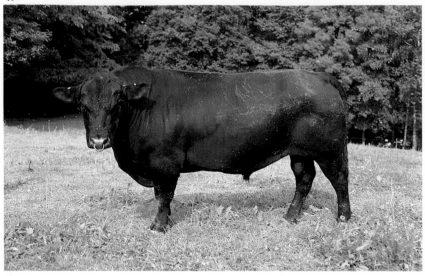

Aberdeen Angus

Characteristics: In conformation it is the most distinctive beef cattle breed. Small-framed. Completely black (in North and South America there is also a reddish brown strain, the Red Angus). Short-legged. Deep torso. The body is barrel-shaped and quite rectangular. The breast bone projects clearly between the front legs. Small, short head. Polled.

	Bull	Cow
Height at shoulder	130	120
Weight	800–900	450–550

Distribution: UK. North and South America. New Zealand. Australia. Germany.

Uses: Resistant to harsh weather. Markedly good-natured and placid. Undemanding. Adaptable. High carcase yield. Fine-fibred, nicely marbled meat. The golden colour of the fat is typical of the breed. The average daily weight gain on fattening test stations is about 1150 g. Above 350 kg live weight a lot of fat is laid down. Matures extremely early. Calves easily. Good rearing ability. Hornlessness is passed on as a dominant characteristic.

Breed history: The breed arose in north-east Scotland in the counties of Aberdeen and Angus. Excavations have revealed that polled cattle existed there in prehistoric times. Deliberate breeding began at the end of the eighteenth century. The breeder H. Watson has rendered great service to the development of the breed. The first herd book was published in 1862. The first animals were exported to the USA and other countries in 1878.

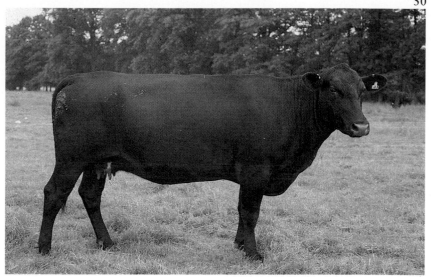

German Angus

Characteristics: Medium-framed beef cattle. There are two colour types, black to dark brown, and red to golden-grey, which are however recorded in the same herd book. There may be white markings. Barrel-shaped. Long body. Good muscle formation on haunches, loins and shoulders. Firm udder with short strokes. Polled characteristic must be inherited for entry into the herd book.

	Bull	Cow
Height at shoulder	130–140	125–130
Weight	1000–1200	500–700

Distribution: Germany; there is no cohesive breeding area.
Uses: Good mothers. Contented. Adaptable. All animals good-natured, including old bulls. Good rearing and fattening characteristics. Daily weight gain on fattening test stations about 1300g for bulls. The selling weight of 10-month-old bull calves is about 300–400kg; female calves weigh about 50kg less at this age. High carcase yield. Excellent meat quality. Mature early. Age of first calving is 24–27 months. Calve easily.
Breed history: Developed in Germany in the 1960s by combination crossing involving Aberdeen Angus and German dual-purpose breeds (mainly Friesian, Golden and Spotted). Now quite uniform in type.

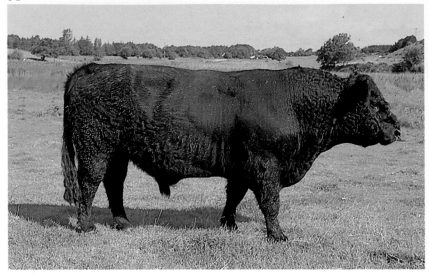

Galloway

Characteristics: The breed is small- to medium-framed. The hair is long, soft and wavy with a thick undercoat. The most common colour is black, and there are also yellowish-grey to light brown animals; white ones are rare. New-born calves are mahogany brown. The Belted Galloway, which has a broad, white band around the middle of the body, is kept as a separate breed. The head is short and broad, the ears are of medium length and wide, and are fringed with long hair. The neck is of medium length, the shoulders are angular and high; the brisket is full and deep. The rear haunches are well-covered, but round haunches are undesirable. Longer than, but not so deep as the Aberdeen Angus. Polled.

Distribution: UK, mainly Scotland. Growing demand in Canada, Argentina, Australia, the former Soviet Union and other countries. Germany since the start of the 1970s.

Uses: Undemanding with respect to fodder and husbandry. Hardy. Quiet temperament, placid and obedient. Suited to crossing with other breeds, traditionally with the Shorthorn. Good-quality meat, tender and well-marbled.

Breed history: Has existed for centuries in the Galloway region of south-west Scotland. Oldest cattle breed in UK. Unfortunately, all records of the breed were destroyed in a fire in 1851. The breed society was formed in 1878; the first Galloway herd book was published a year later. No other breeds have ever been crossed with it.

	Bull	Cow
Height at shoulder	128	120
Weight	800	450–500

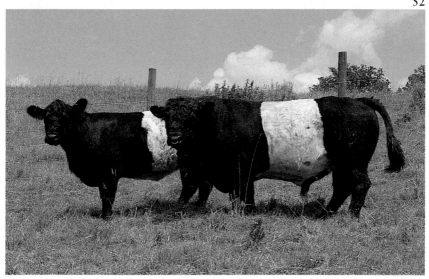

Belted Galloway

Characteristics: Medium- to small-framed beef cattle. Broad, flat head. Neck is of medium length. Deep torso. Well-rounded brisket. Short, clean legs. Fine bone structure. Thick, soft, long hair, especially in winter. The fore- and hind-quarters are black with a reddish sheen; the middle of the body is white. Occasionally there are brown animals. Polled.

	Bull	Cow
Height at shoulder	128	120
Weight	750–950	500–600

Distribution: UK, USA, Canada, New Zealand, Argentina and some African states. In Germany, there are famous populations mainly north of Frankfurt and at Pfaffenhofen.
Uses: Hardy. Undemanding. Adaptable. Good-natured and easily controlled. Outstanding meat quality. Well suited to all-purpose crossing. Hornlessness is inherited as a dominant characteristic. Calve easily. Cows are good mothers.
Breed history: The 'Belties', like six other colour variants, presumably originated centuries ago in the pure black Galloways. They were mentioned as early as the start of the last century. It is assumed that other belted breeds were crossed with them, but there is no proof of this. In 1921 several breeders formed a society. In 1922 an independent herd book was established for this breed. It contained 200 animals at that time. After World War II numerous populations were built up again in the UK. This breed has been familiar on the continent of Europe since about 1970. An independent breed society was founded in North America in 1951; a corresponding society in New Zealand is concerned with both pure black and Belted Galloway cattle.

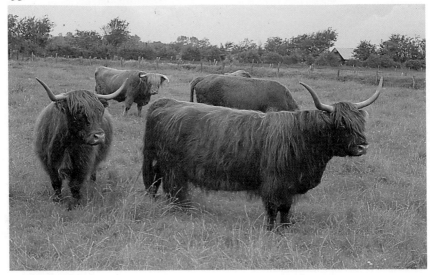

Scottish Highland Cattle, Highlands

Characteristics: Small-framed. Generally they are reddish brown or golden all over; rarely black, white or spotted. Long, shaggy hair. Short, broad head. Long horns, curving out and up. Short legs.

	Bull	Cow
Height at shoulder	125–130	110–120
Weight	500–600	400–450

The Kyloe breed in the west of Scotland is somewhat smaller.

Distribution: Originally west and central Scotland and the Hebrides. For some years they have been in numerous herds in central and northern Europe as well as North America.

Uses: Robust, tolerant of severe weather, undemanding, long-lived. Suitable for use as suckler cows. Mature late. Good as wet-nurses. Top-quality meat.

Breed history: Original cattle of the western Highlands of Scotland and the outlying islands. Since deliberate cattle breeding has been carried out in the UK for about 200 years, this breed has existed unchanged and without being crossed with other breeds. The Highland Cattle Breed Society was founded in 1884; the first herd book animals were registered in 1885. The Verband Deutscher Highland Cattle-Züchter und -Halter e.V. (Association of German Highland Cattle Breeders and Farmers) was founded in Germany in 1983. Currently there are almost 100 breeders and farmers in Germany with a total of about 500 cows.

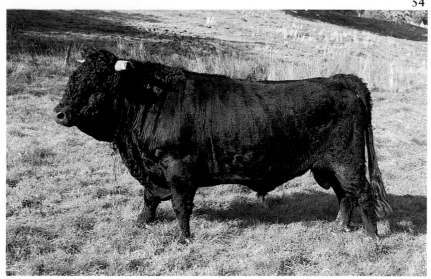

Dexter

Characteristics: Extremely small cattle. Broad, deep torso. Very short legs with noticeably angled back legs. Heavily muscled hind-quarters. Well-developed udder. Usually black, sometimes brown (cow) or dark red (bull). The horns are upturned.

	Bull	Cow
Height at shoulder	115	100–110
Weight	400–450	300–350

Distribution: Numerous small herds in the UK and a few other countries. In Germany there are populations in the Taunus and in the Hamburg region.
Uses: Dual-purpose breed with a remarkable annual milk yield for their size of on average 2500 kg (4.3% fat). Some cows achieve an annual milk yield which is 20 times their body weight. Undemanding and long-lived.

There is a high proportion of malformed calves (bulldog calves), which are aborted between the fifth and ninth months of pregnancy.
Breed history: This breed is regarded as a dwarf strain of the Irish Kerry. It was developed in the south-west of Ireland at the end of the eighteenth century by Mr Dexter who wanted to breed a small animal that would be suitable for dairy and beef purposes. Mr Dexter had a very small, short-legged cow with a large udder covered by a Kerry bull. The offspring were the basis of the breed. It is no longer kept in Ireland. It was introduced into the UK in 1882. In 1905 the Dexter Cattle Society was founded. This breed has a population size which makes it endangered; for this reason, semen from several bulls has been deep frozen as a gene reserve.

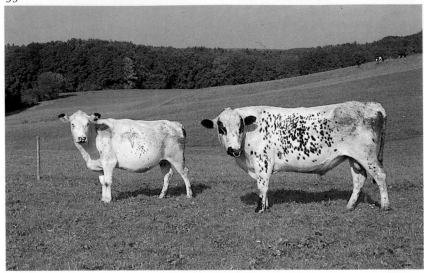

Fjäll

Characteristics: Small, dainty cattle with a fine bone structure and distinct dairy conformation. Good body depth. Well-developed udder. The colour varies from white with just a few dark spots to almost complete pigmentation with only a little white. The pigment is either red or black. At least the ears and area around the eyes as well as the muzzle are pigmented. When there is heavy pigmentation the colour pattern resembles that of the Vosges and the Pustertal Spotted. Fjäll cattle belong to one of the few naturally hornless breeds.

	Bull	Cow
Height at shoulder	128	120
Weight	600	380–420

Distribution: Sweden. Similar hornless breeds, with which there are blood links, in Norway (Black-sided Trondheim) and Finland (North Finnish). There is quite a sizeable population in eastern Germany.

Uses: Robust. Well suited to a harsh climate. Lively and good-natured. Exceedingly prolific. Long-lived. The annual milk yield is approximately 4000 kg (4.2% fat).

Breed history: There is evidence that considerable numbers of hornless cattle have lived in Scandinavia for many centuries. These animals aroused great interest from the end of the nineteenth century onwards. There were two types: one predominantly red and one mainly white. The two were combined in one herd book in 1938, yet there was scarcely any exchange of blood between the two types afterwards. There is close breeding contact with corresponding breeds in neighbouring countries. The number of animals is falling, and the population is endangered.

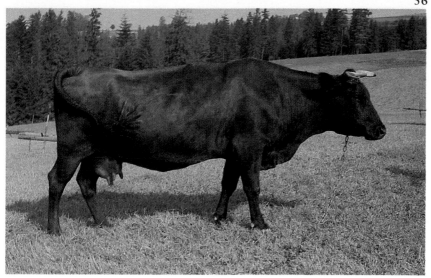

Polish Red

Characteristics: Medium-sized. Mono-coloured, cherry to brownish red. Head, neck, belly and legs are often darker than the rest of the body. Broad head of medium length. Straight back. Sloping pelvis. Moderate muscling. Small udder covered in fine hair. Short horns; in the cow they curve sharply forwards.

	Bull	Cow
Height at shoulder	132–138	122–128
Weight	700–900	400–550

Distribution: North-east, south and south-east Poland. Kept mainly in small holdings.
Uses: Robust. Long-lived. Contented. Willing draught animals. Very prolific. Milk yield of pure-bred Polish Red on average 2600 kg per year. Milk has a high fat (4.1%) and protein (3.5%) content. Calf losses are low.

Breed history: Selective breeding was carried out by societies founded at the end of the last century. Subsequently, East Friesian Red and Shorthorn were increasingly crossed with Polish Red. From 1910 and especially after World War II, Red Danish bulls were imported. Since 1978, several thousand semen doses from Angeln bulls have been imported. To prevent the Polish Red dying out, a preserve was created at Nowy Sacz in 1975. There is a performance test station for young Red bulls and a progeny test station for milk yield characteristics. The total population of cows is about 200,000, 3% of the Polish cattle population. Angeln and other Red cattle breeds have recently been crossed with a large part of the population. In three holdings the original Polish Red is kept as a gene reserve to preserve the breed.

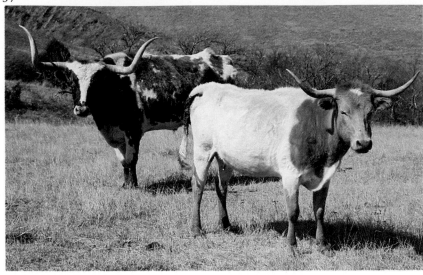

Texas Longhorn

Characteristics: Small, slim cattle. Very variable colouring. An individual animal may have areas of black, grey, brown and white. There are examples which are mono-coloured, or have patches, spots or brindling. They are long-legged, slim and lightly muscled. The horns are impressively long and spreading, especially in old oxen.

	Bull	Cow
Height at shoulder	130	120
Weight	600	350–400

Distribution: North America, especially the south-west USA and north Mexico. **Uses:** Undemanding. Robust. Suitable for arid regions. Temperamental. Prepared to resist larger predators. Can be used for crossing programmes and for initial serving of heifers of other breeds. Dry, lean meat, suitable for many specialities.

Breed history: It was brought by the Spanish via Mexico into the territory of the modern USA in the sixteenth century. With intense settlement of the south west it spread to the north east of the USA. After the American Civil War (1861–65) there was an explosive increase in the population. Animals intended for slaughter were driven slowly along the wide 'trails', taking two years to reach market in the more densely populated north east of the USA. In the extremely hard winter of 1885/86, about 85% of the animals died in some areas. After the subsequent extremely dry summer and an unusually severe blizzard in January 1887, holdings completely collapsed and the importance of this breed was practically destroyed. In the 1920s there were only a few hundred Longhorns remaining. The population has been built up again with government help, and is now about 8000.

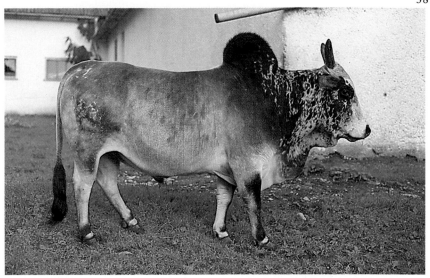

Dwarf Zebu

Characteristics: Dainty cattle with a hump at the withers. There are black, grey, brown, and white animals as well as some with patches and brindling. Slim. Often with shortened pelvis. Long legs. Horns set high and pointing up or back. Lop ears. Large dewlap. Pronounced foreskin.

	Bull	*Cow*
Height at shoulder	120	110–115
Weight	250–300	200

Distribution: Sri Lanka, Caucasus, East Africa, Thailand and other countries. In Germany there is one large herd and several small ones and individual animals are kept as a hobby.
Uses: Resistant to high temperatures. Immune to many tropical diseases. Undemanding. Suitable for extensive rearing.

Breed history: The word 'zebu' is derived from the Tibetan word 'ceba', which means 'hump'. Zebus, like European domestic cattle, are descended from the aurochs. The earliest bones found with typical Zebu characteristics date back to the third millenium BC. It appears that they were developed in the Middle East soon after cattle were domesticated. Their area of distribution subsequently extended from China to West Africa. Zebus are adapted to tropical and sub-tropical conditions. For this reason they are now kept in similar regions of America. Interbreeding with breeds of European origin occurring from the southern USA to the north of Argentina and in South Africa has proved particularly advantageous. Dwarf Zebus have been kept successfully in Germany for some years as herds of suckler cows.

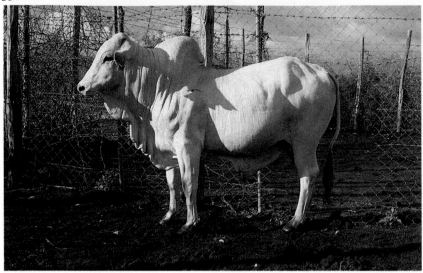

Boran

Characteristics: Medium-framed. A breast-hump type of cattle. Fairly long head with a broad forehead. Slightly lop ears. Powerful, well-muscled body. Slightly heavy build. Good depth to body. Sloping pelvis, tail set low. Dewlap extends down between front legs. Very pendulous foreskin. The most common colour is white, but there are also golden, brown, grey and (rarely) black and patterned animals. The bull shown has been polled; there are, however, also naturally hornless animals.

	Bull	*Cow*
Height at shoulder	125	120 ·
Weight	550–675	400–475

Distribution: Originally South Ethiopia and the neighbouring parts of Somalia and northern Kenya. Now also distributed over other areas of East Africa. Small numbers in Zaire.

Uses: Well-suited to hot, dry regions. The improved Boran Zebu of Kenya is a beef animal, but is also used for draught. The cows are sometimes milked. Good-quality meat. One of the most productive local African breeds, which compares well with European beef breeds in the given conditions.

Breed history: The Boran was originally bred from the stock of the Borana on the Liban plateau in South Ethiopia. In the 1920s and 1930s this breed was brought primarily to the dry regions of Kenya by Somali merchants. There it was bred selectively for beef (Improved Boran). It is assumed that European beef breeds (e.g. Hereford) were crossed with them. In recent decades, Charolais and other European beef breeds have been crossed with them, as have Zebus from the Middle East and America.

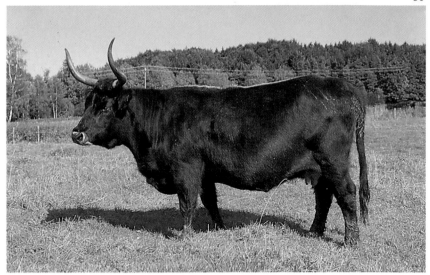

New Aurochs

Characteristics: Bulls are black with golden line-back. Cows are reddish brown with a darker neck. The area around the muzzle is white in both sexes. In summer the hair is silky-smooth and short; in winter it is longer and coarser. Older animals have long, powerful, forward-sweeping horns. The calves are born light brown.

	Bull	Cow
Height at shoulder	140	130
Weight	750	550

Distribution: Germany, Austria and Switzerland. Mainly in zoological gardens, but also in agricultural enterprises.
Uses: Resistant to harsh weather. Contented cattle. They have increasingly been kept for landscape tending and beef production in recent years. As the cow always rears her calf herself, the milk yield is unknown. Largely disease-resistant.

Breed history: At the end of the 1920s, the 'Aurochs makers' Heinz and Lutz Heck tried to recreate the extinct Aurochs in the zoos of Munich and Berlin by crossing domestic breeds of cattle. Heinz Heck crossed Hungarian Steppe, Scottish Highland, Brown, Murnau-Werdenfels, Angeln and Lowland Friesian (now German Friesian) with one another. Later the Podolic and the Corsican were crossed with them. In Berlin, Lutz Heck crossed Spanish and French fighting cattle with other breeds. The results of the two breeders were largely similar. The Berlin breed later failed, so today's animals are descended only from the Hellabrunn breed. These cattle are now quite uniform in conformation and have been largely uninfluenced by outside blood in recent years. The total population is about 150 animals.

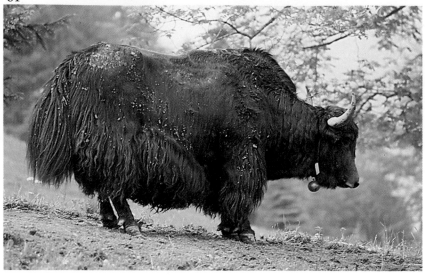

Yak

Characteristics: In addition to black, various shades of brown, grey and white, there are also patterned animals, usually with blazes on the back. The area around the mouth is always pale. The torso is covered with long hair, and there is an extremely prominent belly mane. The whole length of the tail is covered in long hair. The mouth is completely covered in hair. Yaks therefore have no muzzle. High, humped shoulders. Powerful, very hairy, short limbs. Spreading horns, but occasionally also hornless.

	Bull	Cow
Height at shoulder	112–120	107–112
Weight	300–400	250–280

Distribution: The wild form in Tibet is almost extinct; domesticated form in China, Nepal, Kashmir, Bhutan, Mongolia, Siberia and North America.

Isolated animals in other countries. Small groups in the Alpine regions of Germany, South Tyrol and Switzerland, sometimes interbred with other types of cattle. Otherwise, kept only as individual animals or for non-commercial reasons.

Uses: Mature late. Long-lived. Kept on land between 300 and 6000 m above sea level. Annual milk yield about 400 kg (7% fat). Milk is made into butter, cheese or sour milk. The meat is cut into strips and dried around the cooking fire and smoked. The annual fleece gives about 3 kg of raw wool, which is made into blankets, tent fabric and rope. In the Himalayas, the dried dung is used as fuel. Used for riding and as beasts of burden, carrying loads of up to 100 kg. The Tibetan civilisation is largely dependent on Yak keeping.

Breed history: Domesticated at least 3000 years ago. On the fringes of the range they are often crossed with domestic cattle.

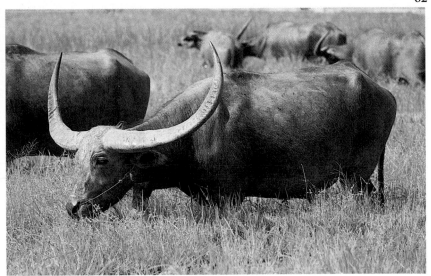

Domestic Buffalo

Characteristics: Massive build. Deep, barrel-shaped body. Sparse hair. Long, narrow head. Slightly domed forehead. Straight back. Powerful hind-quarters. Sloping pelvis. Tail is low-set. Relatively short legs. Grey to black, occasionally tending towards brown. There may be white markings; occasionally there are pure-white animals. Horned. The horns of all buffalo are triangular in section. They either turn down to the side of the head and then up in an arc (curly) or sweep back in a sickle shape.

	Bull	Cow
Height at shoulder	125–145	120–140
Weight	500–900	350–600

Distribution: South and East Asia, Egypt, the Balkans, the former Soviet Republics and Brazil.
Uses: There are many different breeds which have been developed for various purposes. The best known application for domestic buffalo is probably as draught animals in rice-growing areas. In Indonesia there is a breed which is kept for fighting. On Bali, domestic buffalo are used for cart racing. In the north west of India and in Europe buffalo are kept mainly for their milk. The annual milk yield of good cows, depending on breed, is between 1500 and 3000kg (7–8% fat). Domestic buffalo in human care are placid and patient, and also easy to control.
Breed history: Domestication is assumed to have started 3000 years BC. They have existed in Europe since the sixth century. There are 130 million domestic buffalo world-wide, with the largest populations in India (64.5 million), China (19.5 million) and Pakistan (13.0 million). European countries that keep buffalo include Italy (one million), Hungary (several hundred) and Yugoslavia (41,000).

Sheep

Of the larger agricultural livestock, sheep are almost as numerous as cattle world-wide. There are three reasons for this:

- No religious taboo.
- Wide range of uses.
- Extreme adaptability.

There is no religious community or culture in the world that forbids the killing of sheep and the consumption of sheep meat. Sheep provide not only meat and wool; some breeds give a lot of milk, which is sold fresh or made into cheese and other products. Strings made from the muscle layer of the small intestine of sheep are of considerable value to some developing countries as foreign currency earners.

Sheep can adapt well to varied climatic and geographical conditions. They are found from the as yet undyked foreshore of the North Sea coast to high mountains and from areas within the polar circles to the tropics. Sheep utilise above all the extensive steppes and semi-deserts of the earth (65). In central Europe they are frequently kept on marginal land, which is unsuitable for cattle and other livestock. As they are good-natured, they can graze with cattle and horses. This does not reduce the stocking rate for the larger animals, as sheep have a different grazing spectrum. In recent years they have frequently been used for landscape maintenance in the German-speaking countries. Their grazing protects heath, moor and high pasture from becoming overgrown. The way in which they eat – sheep grasp the food with their teeth and bite the grass off just above the ground – and the uniform loading of the ground by their 'golden hooves', have a protective effect on the pasture and give a good sward. The famous lawns of England can apparently be traced back to this influence. In areas of intensive agricultural use, sheep sometimes feed extensively on harvest remnants.

In the past, sheep were kept in central Europe and other areas primarily for wool. The importance of wool has fallen sharply since the development of synthetic fibres, although it is essential for making the best fabrics. Merino sheep give the finest wool. The long- and short-wool breeds give coarser wool. This is also processed into fabrics. Half of all sheep in the world have wool which is so coarse that it cannot be used for clothing, only for carpets and blankets. These breeds are a minority here, however. Examples of these are the German Heath and the

Karakul. In the tropics, i.e. in areas of high temperatures and high humidity, there is a large proportion of Hairy sheep. Instead of wool, they have hair, and moult twice a year like other animal species. Their hair can be regarded as a necessary adaptation to the climate of the regions in such native breeds. In Europe, the only Hairy sheep are imports from more southerly areas. In Germany, there are some attempts to cross Hairy sheep with indigenous breeds to create animals which are suitable for the tropics while producing more meat.

There is great breed diversity among sheep. The reason for this is that in general sheep are still kept in extensive stocking systems. Special features of food and climate produce local breeds which can scarcely be replaced with another. In Germany there is no breed better suited to the ground and the vegetation of the heath than the Grey Horned Heath, and none is so at home on the soft marshland and knows how to utilise the special, sparse plant life of the moor better than the Marsh. Thus the sheep population is assured in relatively untouched areas such as marsh and heath, so long as no other factors intervene. In the past, sheep in central Europe – apart from in areas such as marsh and mountain – were tended by a shepherd in the open countryside. The sheep had to have certain characteristics for this type of husbandry: long legs for an extensive stride; hard, disease-resistant hooves; and not too high a body-weight. The decline of free-range sheep keeping because of increasing traffic density, more intensive utilisation of agricultural land and other commercial factors, forced a change in sheep husbandry methods. Today, a large number of sheep are kept in enclosures, and are not supervised continuously. This trend has brought sheep back into the farmyard in smaller populations. These animals therefore do not have to cover great distances every day. On the contrary: a tendency to wander is undesirable; it means that animals escape. This has meant that breeds suited to free-range farming have in some cases been modified and that breeds suitable for keeping in enclosures are increasingly being kept. This tendency is being countered by another trend: the sheep farmer today earns over 90% of his income from the meat. The consequence is that animals are bred to put on more meat, or the indigenous *meat* breeds are kept more often, and other such breeds are imported into central Europe. Meat breeds are as a rule more phlegmatic than wool breeds and land races and hence are better suited to living in enclosures.

Sheep breeds are usually divided into wool, meat, and land races. This classification scarcely corresponds to the actual situation. This is not just because, for example, the Mutton Merino – the breed with the finest wool in West Germany – can be assigned to two categories, i.e. it is basically a dual-purpose sheep. Milk sheep, with their enormous milk yields, which can be ten times their bodyweight, have achieved a

63

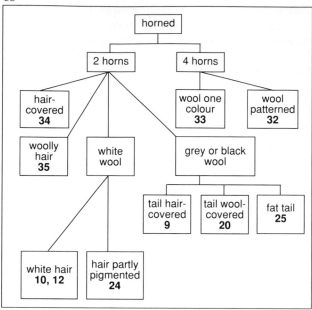

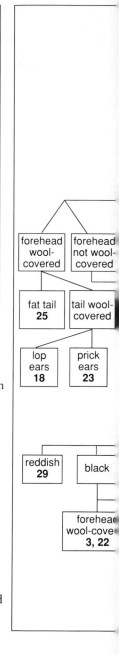

63, 64 Key for the identification of sheep breeds by easily recognisable features.

1 = Merino Land
2 = Mutton Merino
3 = Black–headed Mutton
4 = White-headed Mutton
5 = Texel
6 = East Friesland Milk (white)
7 = Black Milk
8 = Leine
9 = Grey Horned Heath
10 = White Horned Heath
11 = Moor
12 = Skudde
13 = Rough-woolled Pomeranian Land
14 = Bentheim Land
15 = Rhön
16 = Coburg Fox
17 = White Mountain
18 = Brown Mountain
19 = Carinthian Spectacled

20 = Stone
21 = White Alpine
22 = Brown–headed Mutton
23 = Black–Brown Mountain
24 = Valais Black–nosed
25 = Karakul
26 = Romanov
27 = Suffolk
28 = Blue–headed Mutton (Bleu de Maine)
29 = Charollais
30 = Flemish
31 = Finnish
32 = Jacob
33 = St. Kilda
34 = Cameroon
35 = Soay
36 = Black–Brown–Woolled form of the Blue–headed Mutton

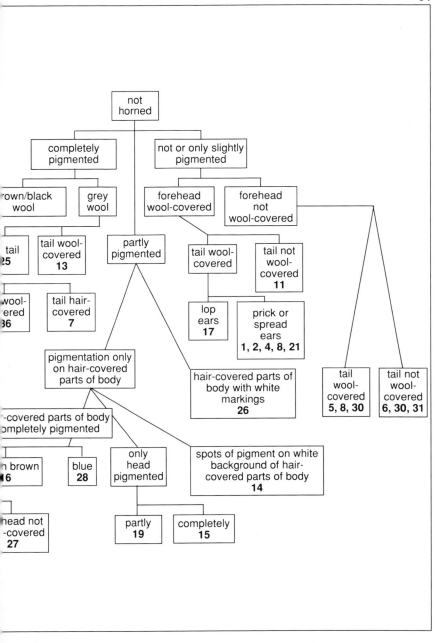

Table 8. Sheep population of the former Federal Republic of Germany by breed.

Breed	1955*		1968		1985	
	No.	%	No.	%	No.	%
Merino Land	514,066	43.3	332,939	40.2	541,084	41.7
Black-hd. Mutton	315,896	26.6	231,719	28.0	324,200	24.9
Texel	–	–	33,071	4.0	114,224	8.8
White-hd. Mutton	112,905	9.5	109,296	13.2	97,165	7.5
Heath	30,170	2.5	11,574	1.4	26,315	2.1
Mutton Merino	114,888	9.7	59,996	7.2	13,012	1.0
Mountain	5,468	0.5	7,500	0.9	24,150	1.9
Milk	56,795	4.8	25,276	3.1	22,056	1.7
Rhön	3,721	0.3	2,706	0.3	8,203	0.6
Bentheim Land	2,497	0.2	1,500	0.2	400	0.0
Blue hd. Mutton	–	–	–	–	3,672	0.3
Leine	23,133	2.0	881	0.1	1,000	0.1
Karakul	466	0.0	100	0.0	80	0.0
Others	8,038	0.7	12,155	1.5	3,742	0.3
Crosses					118,113	9.1
Total	1,188,043		828,713		1,297,516	

*Before 1955 no details of individual breeds available. Source: Business reports of Vereinigung Deutscher Landesschafzuchtverbände (Association of German Regional Sheep Breed Societies) et al.

Table 9. Total sheep population of Austria by individual breed, 1979.

Breed	No.	%
Mountain	151,200	77.4
Texel	11,000	5.6
Black-hd.	10,500	5.4
Milk	1,300	0.7
Stone	400	0.2
Karakul	400	0.2
Others + crosses	20,600	10.5

Table 10. Distribution of flock book animals among individual sheep breeds in Switzerland, 1984.

Breed	No.	%
White Alpine	43,640	60.6
Brown-hd. Mutton	10,801	15.0
Black-Brown Mutton	6,722	9.3
Valais Black-nosed	10,874	15.1

Source: 1984 Annual Report of Schweiz. Zentralstelle für Kleinviehzucht (Swiss Central Office for Small Livestock Breeding).

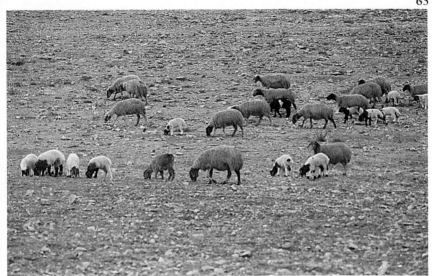

65   Sheep in the Negev, Israel.

specialisation which no longer corresponds to the term 'land sheep'. Owing to their special husbandry and feeding, and the fact that they are strongly fixated on man, milk sheep occupy a special position. Land races have their own advantages. Their grazing maintains the structure of the landscape and they make their mark on it. After a temporary decline, the land races have increased in importance for this reason and, not least, because it has been recognised that old breeds are a cultural asset.

In Austria, mountain sheep form the greater part of the total population (**Table 9**). The Stone (Steinschaf) is worthy of mention as an indigenous breed which is increasing in numbers. The remaining breeds have been imported in recent decades.

In Switzerland, too, one breed is dominant – the White Alpine (**Table 10**). The Valais Black-nosed is of purely local significance.

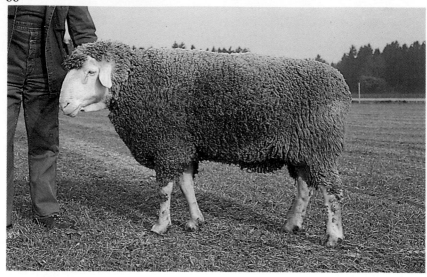

Merino Land

Characteristics: Medium- to large-framed. Parts of body covered with wool and hair are white. Head is of medium length, not too broad. Long, broad ears hanging slightly towards the front. Forehead and corner of lower jaw wool-covered. Straight, broad back. Good depth to breast and flanks. As a free-range animal it used to have long legs for a long stride. Today they tend to have shorter legs. Emphasis is increasingly laid on improving the loin formation. Polled.

	Ram	Ewe
Height at shoulder	90–100	75–85
Weight	120–140	80–90

Distribution: South Germany.
Uses: Sheep capable of walking but also suited to living in enclosures. Robust. Lambs suitable for fattening.

Wool of merino type. Annual fleece yield of ewes 4.0–5.0 kg ewes. Reproduction aseasonal.

Breed history: In the middle of the eighteenth century, fine-woolled sheep came to Germany from Spain. Sheep of this type were used to improve land race sheep in south Germany at the end of the eighteenth century, especially in Württemberg. In 1887 this south German white-headed sheep appeared at the first DLG exhibition as a specific breed. The subsequent crossing of more Merinos then led to the 'Württemberg', a name which has been gradually replaced with the modern name since 1906. Bred deliberately for wool and for meat. 'Württemberg' or Merino Land sheep have been crossed into the White Alpine sheep of Switzerland and other breeds.

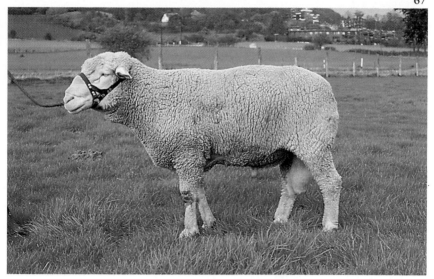

Mutton Merino

Characteristics: Medium-sized animals with a wide, deep torso. Pure white, skin on face white. Bridge of nose slightly domed. Wool extends to eye-line. The medium-length legs have wool down to the carpal and tarsal joints. Polled.

	Ram	Ewe
Height at shoulder	80–90	75–85
Weight	120–140	75–85

Distribution: In the former Federal Republic of Germany, almost exclusively in Lower Saxony. Still highly regarded in other countries, especially in the Eastern Bloc. Has been exported to Turkey, South Africa and South America.

Uses: Easy to feed; robust. Grows fast and puts meat on easily. Carcase yield 48–50%. Top wool quality of all German breeds. Annual fleece yield 4.5–5.0 kg (ewes), 6.0–7.0 kg (rams). Good fertility. Lambing percentage 150–220%.

Breed history: Merino sheep originated in Spain. The name is derived from the Berber line of the Beri–Merines, who came from North Africa to Spain in the twelfth century and brought the ancestors of the Merinos with them. The first Merinos arrived in Germany in the eighteenth century. The modern Mutton Merino was developed in the nineteenth century from German Merinos by crossing with French Merino Combing Wool sheep and English meat breeds. It was distributed mainly in the area to the east of the Elbe. The population has fallen considerably in recent years. There are now about 24,000 animals.

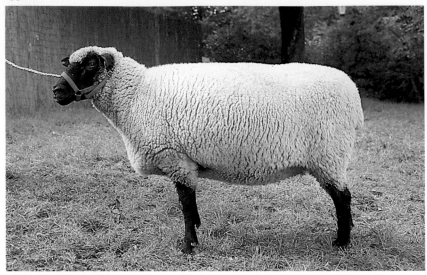

Black-headed Mutton

Characteristics: Medium build. Wool white. Head and legs from front knee and hock down are black or dark brown. Forehead wool-covered. Head of medium length. Strong ears extending to the sides. Deep brisket, long back, good loin formation. Polled.

	Ram	Ewe
Height at		
shoulder	80–90	75–80
Weight	100–130	70–90

Distribution: North and west Germany. In recent years, increasingly in Bavaria and Austria.
Uses: Suitable for enclosed and free-range husbandry. Meat sheep. Very good carcase quality. Rams are used in flocks of other breeds for producing marked crossed lambs. Annual fleece yield 4.0–5.0 kg (ewes), 5.0–7.0 kg (rams). Mature early. Seasonal reproduction, but long covering season. Lambing percentage 120–170%.
Breed history: Originates essentially in English meat sheep breeds (Hampshire, Oxford, Suffolk), which were imported into Germany from 1870. The reason was the fall in the price of wool and an increase in the significance of meat production. In Germany it quickly spread in areas with a maritime climate. Initially, the English breeds mentioned were separate. During World War I they were combined to form one breed.

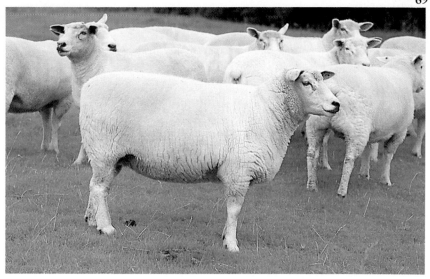

White-headed Mutton

Characteristics: Large frame, good muscling. Body parts covered with wool and hair are always pure white. Mucous membranes of nose have dark pigmentation. Forehead is wool-covered. Medium-sized ears standing out to the sides. Deep, broad and long ('barrel-shaped') body. Loins well developed. Polled.

	Ram	Ewe
Height at		
shoulder	75–85	70–90
Weight	110–130	80–90

Distribution: Almost exclusive to Schleswig–Holstein and Lower Saxony. Mainly on the coast.

Uses: Good fodder utilisation. Robust. Hardy in winter conditions. Well suited to living in enclosures. Put on meat fast. Good carcase quality. Crossbred wool. Annual fleece yield 5.0–6.5 kg (ewes), 6.0–7.0 kg (rams). Mature early. Seasonal reproduction. Lambing percentage 150–180%.

Breed history: Developed in the nineteenth century from the indigenous Marsh sheep of the North Sea coast by crossing with various British meat sheep breeds and Texel sheep. Recognised as an independent breed since 1924. Breeding aimed to produce a white, early-maturing, heavy-fleeced sheep with a good body shape and strong bone structure. In recent years, Texel sheep have frequently been used for crossing.

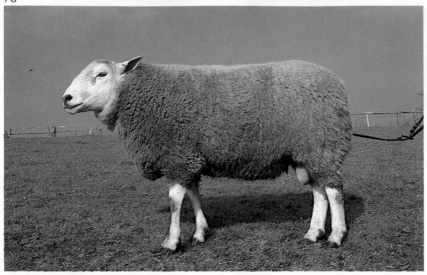

Texel

Characteristics: Medium to large build. Body parts with and without wool are white. Flecks of pigment often visible through the skin of the ears. Head of medium length, broad and flat. Strong prick ears of medium length. Neck short and well muscled. Deep brisket, broad back. Full loins, extending a long way down. Strong leg bones. Relatively short legs. Polled.

	Ram	Ewe
Height at shoulder	75–80	70–75
Weight	110–130	70–90

Distribution: Central and eastern Europe, but also South America, Africa and southern Asia.
Uses: Particularly well suited for keeping in enclosures. Markedly a meat sheep. Lambs grow fast. Daily weight gains of 400 g are not unusual. Annual fleece yield 4.0–5.0 kg (ewes), 5.0–6.0 kg (rams). Mature early. Seasonal reproduction. Lambing percentage 150–200%.

Breed history: Originated on the Netherlands island of Texel, where it is said to have developed from long-legged sheep brought by seafarers from the east coast of Africa. Subsequently distributed over the whole of the Netherlands, where it is now by far the most common sheep breed. In the middle of the nineteenth century English meat breeds were crossed with it. From the start of the 1960s it was imported into the former Federal Republic of Germany, initially to north Germany, and later to south Germany.

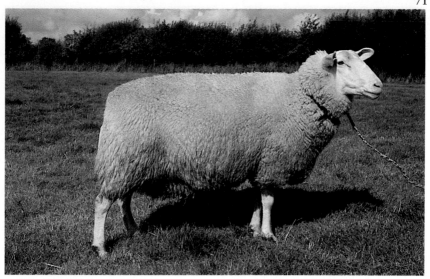

East Friesland Milk

Characteristics: Large build. White longwool sheep. For a long time there have been occasional black animals. The longish head with a slightly depressed nose is free of wool and has only fine spiky hairs. Long ears pointing forwards. The tail is long, thin and has no wool. Polled.

	Ram	*Ewe*
Height at shoulder	80–90	70–80
Weight	110–130	80–100

Distribution: Occurs over the whole of Germany, Austria and Switzerland as well as in many other countries. The breed is centred on North-Rhine/ Westphalia and the Weser-Ems region.
Uses: Unlike other sheep breeds, the milk sheep is not a flock animal. It is particularly suited to keeping in enclosures. Annual fleece yield 4.5– 5.0 kg (ewes), 5.5–6.0 kg (rams). Average annual milk yield 600 kg (5.5% fat); peak yields of over 1400 kg (over 6% fat). Lambing percentage 230%. First lambing is possible at 12 months. Mature early, prolific, fast-growing. Seasonal rutting.
Breed history: It was mentioned in the sixteenth century as being exceptionally prolific. Originally native to East Friesland. Later, especially in hard times, valued like the goat as the 'small man's cow'. Planned flock book breed since 1908. Exported to many countries where ewe's milk is valued.

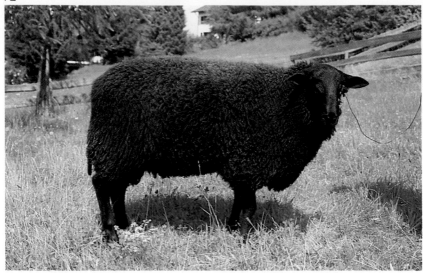

Black Milk

Characteristics: Somewhat lighter than the East Friesian Milk sheep, otherwise similar in shape and type. Uniformly brown to deep black without markings. The lambs are born black. The head has fine hairs and the nose is slightly depressed. Long, thin ears pointing forwards. Long tail has no wool. Polled.

	Ram	Ewe
Height at shoulder	75–85	70–80
Weight	100–120	80–90

Distribution: Flock book animals kept now only in Baden–Württemberg and Bavaria. They occur in other parts of the former Federal Republic, however.
Uses: Closewool. Annual fleece yield 4.0–4.5 kg (ewes), 5.0–5.5 kg (rams). The annual milk yield of on average little more than 500 kg is about 5%

lower than that of the East Friesian Milk sheep. The breed therefore produces the same amount related to bodyweight. The milk is said to be sweeter and tastier than that of the East Friesian Milk.
Breed history: The predisposition for pigmentation exists recessively in the East Friesian Milk sheep and occasionally expresses itself. In times when there is a special interest in naturally coloured wool – post-war and now – there is a certain demand for black milk sheep. It has been a pure breed for about 20 years.

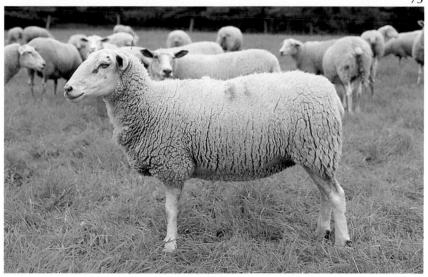

Leine

Characteristics: Large build. White, sometimes with a reddish sheen especially on the head; no flecks of pigment. Long, fine head with sparse hair. The wool starts behind the ears. Long, smooth ears, which tend to hang. Close wool, grows down long. Polled.

	Ram	*Ewe*
Height at shoulder	80–85	70–75
Weight	100–120	70–80

Distribution: Lower Saxony.

Uses: Fast-growing, robust sheep. A good suckler. Undemanding with regard to fodder and husbandry; suited to free-range management as well as living in enclosures. Hardy and adaptable. Good meat yield. Annual fleece yield 3.5–4.0 kg (ewes), 5.0–6.0 kg (rams). First mating at 7–8 months. Seasonal reproduction. Lambing percentage 160–220%.

Breed history: Arose in the 1860s from an old land strain. Crossing with English meat sheep later improved the conformation. There has been a cohesive breeding target since the start of the twentieth century. Cross-breeding in subsequent decades was not successful. Today's Leine sheep is a cross between the original Leine and Texel, Flemish and East Friesian Milk. This has given a combination of the low rate of lambing difficulties and of rearing losses of the old-type Leine with the fertility and high milk yield of the East Friesian Milk and the fast growth rate and high meat percentage of the Texel.

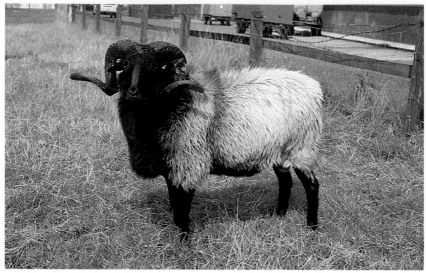

Grey Horned Heath

Characteristics: Light animals with fine limbs. Silver grey to dark grey with a black bib. Rough-woolled. Parts of body without wool (head, tail, legs) are black. The area around the muzzle often has numerous white hairs. The lambs are always born black with curly wool; the wool changes colour during the first year. Older rams have magnificent curly horns which are almost as fine as those of the Mouflon. The ewes have sickle-shaped horns, pointing out and back.

	Ram	*Ewe*
Height at		
shoulder	67	60
Weight	60–70	45–50

Distribution: Originally only the dry, sparse areas of the Lüneburg Heath. In recent years, also the rest of the former Federal Republic of Germany and Switzerland.

Uses: Its grazing of the heather and coniferous growth on the Lüneburg Heath maintains the typical character of the landscape. Undemanding, hardy. Roast Heath lamb is regarded as a delicacy due to its game-like flavour and tenderness. Skins. First mating at the age of about 18 months. Rutting is seasonal.

Breed history: Was kept for centuries without cross-breeding. However, selective breeding since 1921 has given an average weight increase of almost 50%. Since 1848, when the population was nearly 400,000 animals, the number has fallen continuously. Since 1970 there has been a noticeable increase in the breed and distribution beyond the original range.

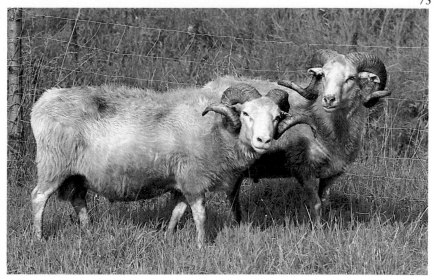

White Horned Heath

Characteristics: Small mixed-wool land sheep. White, no markings. Long, wedge-shaped head with curly horns in the case of rams and sickle-shaped horns curving backwards in the case of ewes. Well-sprung ribs, fine constitution.

	Ram	Ewe
Height at shoulder	55–60	50
Weight	60–75	45–50

Distribution: South Oldenburg, Emsland.

Uses: Contented, hardy, particularly suited to maintenance of heathland. However, it makes more demand on the pasture than the Grey Horned Heath. Outstanding quality meat (tender, game-like flavour). Annual fleece yield 1.8 kg (ewes), 3.5 kg (rams). Good mothers; easy lambing. Lambing percentage 100%.

Breed history: The White Horned Heath is not mentioned in older specialist literature. It is to be assumed that it was developed from the Grey Horned Heath by selective breeding, apparently not until the beginning of the twentieth century. It has survived with the latter for centuries as an original breed without blood from other breeds. In recent decades there has been selection for higher weight; 30 years ago the weight of ewes was about 30–45 kg, and that of rams about 50–60 kg. There is now a total of about 1500 animals.

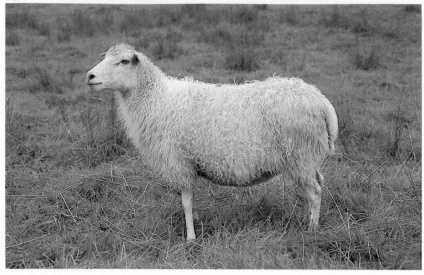

Moor, White Polled Heath

Characteristics: Small, mixed-wool land sheep. Small, longish head with small ears standing up at an angle. Very fine bone structure, firm hooves. Both sexes are polled.

	Ram	Ewe
Height at shoulder	55–60	50
Weight	70–75	40–45

Distribution: Lower Saxony in the vicinity of Diepholz.

Uses: Well adapted to the special conditions of moorland. Very agile. Feeds predominantly on heather, moor grasses and other plants as well as birch shoots. Undemanding and hardy. Particularly suited to free-range husbandry in marshy areas and moors. Meat has game-like taste. First mating at 18 months. Seasonal rutting. Lambing percentage 110%. Weight of fleece 1.7–2.5 kg (ewes), 3.5 kg (rams).

Breed history: Indigenous to the present breeding range for centuries and carefully selected for hardiness and adaptability. Related to other moorland sheep. Only about 100 animals now.

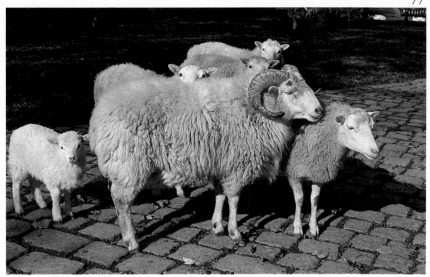

Skudde

Characteristics: Small build. Greyish white, occasionally black or bronzy. Closewool. Relatively large, heavy head. Noticeably small ears. Short tail, lower part hair-covered. Rams have curved horns; female animals have horn stumps or are hornless.

	Ram	Ewe
Height at shoulder	55–60	50
Weight	50–55	40–45

Distribution: Originally East Prussia and the Baltic. Currently a few small flocks in the former Federal Republic of Germany, mainly in Hesse, Saarland and Baden; also some in other parts of the former Federal Republic as well as Berlin and the former German Democratic Republic.

Uses: Tame and undemanding. Good fodder utilisation on sparse pasture.

Hard hooves. Lively but placid. Meat, skins. Annual fleece yield barely 2 kg. The wool is finer than that of similar breeds; it is however only suitable for carpets or coarse loden cloth. A seasonal rutting. Lambing percentage on average 130%. May lamb twice in a year.

Breed history: Long-familiar indigenous land race in region of origin. Belongs to the group of short-tailed, northern heath sheep. The name 'Skudde' is derived from the word 'Kosse', which means 'poor'. After World War I the population declined sharply and was crossed with other sheep breeds. The current population derives essentially from animals which came to south Germany from East Prussia and Lithuania before the end of World War II. Current population: about 600 animals. Valuable genetic reserve.

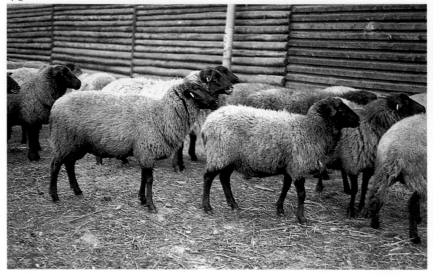

Rough-woolled Pomeranian Land

Characteristics: Mixed-wool land sheep with grey to blue-grey wool with a brownish tinge. Dark, faded 'backline' from the back of the head to the withers. Extremities and head black. Forehead bears some wool. Pale spot before eyes. Old rams may have a black mane extending down to the front of the chest. The lambs are born black. Polled.

	Ram	Ewe
Height at shoulder	70	63
Weight	70–75	50–55

Distribution: The Baltic Sea coast of the former East Germany, mainly on the islands of Rügen and Hiddensee, and on parts of Usedom. In the former West Germany there is only one flock of about 80 sheep as well as a few individual animals. East of the Oder there appear to be only remnants.

Uses: Well suited to meagre grazing conditions (dry, poor sandy ground, moorland, wet meadows), contented and hardy, largely insensitive to bad weather. Resistant to worm diseases and foot rot. Annual fleece yield 4.0 kg (ewes), 6.0 kg (rams). Lambing average 130%.

Breed history: Very old sheep breed. Said to be the result of crossing the former Zaupel with the Hanover. Originally distributed over the German Baltic provinces (Mecklenburg, Pomerania, East Prussia), as well as Silesia and Poland. In many areas the ewes are milked; the milk is used to make cheese. Formerly, widely distributed in Mecklenburg, Pomerania and East Prussia. Population has fallen continuously since the beginning of the nineteenth century. Several attempts at crossing with English meat sheep failed.

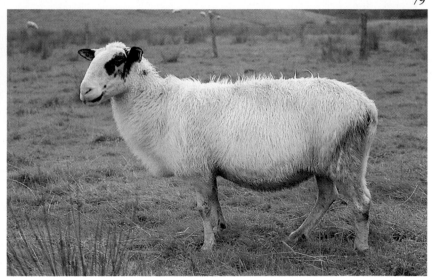

Bentheim Land

Characteristics: Large build, long legs, with long middle hand. The wool is pure white. Dark brown spots on the head and ears as well as on the legs. Long, narrow head. Bridge of nose noticeably compressed. Ears medium to long. Long tail, wool-covered. Polled.

	Ram	*Ewe*
Height at shoulder	70–75	65–70
Weight	80–90	60–70

Distribution: Western Lower Saxony. Small, isolated populations outside this area.

Uses: Hardy. Undemanding. Capable of walking. Hard hooves. Resistant to foot rot. Meat of outstanding quality. Annual fleece yield 4.5–5.0 kg (rams), 3.0–4.0 kg (ewes). First mating possible from 7 months. Good mothers. Excellent sucklers. Lambing percentage 130%.

Breed history: Developed as a result of crossing Dutch animals with native Heath and Marsh. Two factors favoured the import of rams from the Netherlands (especially the Drenthe sheep) and the development of the Bentheim Land. First, the introduction of artifical fertilisers improved pasture productivity, so there was sufficient fodder for heavier sheep; and secondly, heavy, fattened wethers were sold via the Netherlands to Brussels, where there was a good market for such animals. This breed has never been widely distributed. Until recently it was restricted to the regions of Bentheim and Lingen in Emsland. Subjected to developmental breeding since 1934. Ecological changes have largely destroyed its natural moor and heath habitat. Today, the largest flock is outside the original breed area. The population is highly endangered.

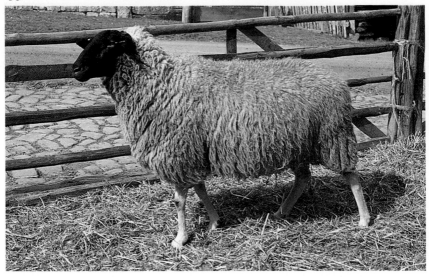

Rhön

Characteristics: Medium to large sheep. White (including the legs). Head is covered with black hair to behind the ears. Slightly compressed nose. Long legs. Closewool. Polled.

	Ram	*Ewe*
Height at shoulder	80–85	72–78
Weight	85–90	60–70

Distribution: Rhön area of Hesse and Bavaria, and its environs. Currently only a few small populations left in the former GDR.

Uses: Suited to the raw, damp climate of the central hill regions. Capable of walking. It is used as a free-range animal as well as in enclosures. The annual fleece yield 3.0–4.0 kg (ewes), 5.0–6.0 kg (rams). First mating at 12–18 months. Aseasonal rutting possible. Good sucklers. Lambing percentage 120%. Fine-tasting meat with a game-like character.

Breed history: First mentioned by name in the literature in 1844, but it is certain that this breed existed considerably earlier. According to the oldest drawing (1873), it already corresponded to the modern type. During the course of time, English Cotswold or Oxfordshire and Merino rams were crossed with it. Since the middle of the nineteenth century, when there were several hundred thousand animals, numbers have fallen continuously, and reached a low point of only 300 registered flock book animals in the former Federal Republic at the end of the 1950s. A definite increase started at the beginning of the 1960s. The population is currently about 1000 animals.

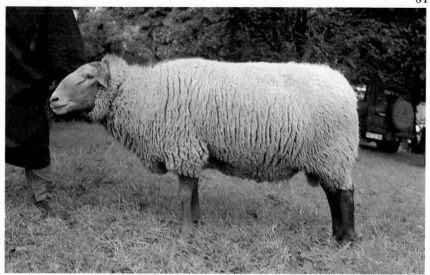

Coburg Fox

Characteristics: Medium-sized. Body parts covered with hair are light to reddish brown. Inside, the fleece has a reddish sheen (golden fleece). Close-wool sheep with a narrow, slightly compressed head. Broad, slightly lop ears. There is no wool on the head to behind the ears, or on the extremities. The lambs are reddish brown up to the age of 6–12 months. Polled.

	Ram	Ewe
Height at shoulder	75–80	60–70
Weight	80–90	55–65

Distribution: Northern Bavaria, isolated flocks in Baden–Württemberg. Fox sheep also occur in France, Italy, Israel and other countries.
Uses: Breed well adapted to the regional conditions. Undemanding and hardy. The dull wool is suitable for making coarse, smooth cloth and fulled fabrics. First mating at 12–18 months. Seasonal rutting. Annual fleece yield 4.5–5.5 kg (rams), 3.5–4.5 kg (ewes). Lambing percentage 140%.
Breed history: Land sheep with foxy colouring have been kept in several regions of Germany for centuries. They almost disappeared as a result of displacement breeding at the beginning of this century. O. Stritzel collected animals typical of the breed from the 1930s onwards. Several foreign breeds were used for crossing. Since 1966 the Coburg Fox has been recognised by the DLG as a breed. Nearly 20 flocks with about 1000 animals.

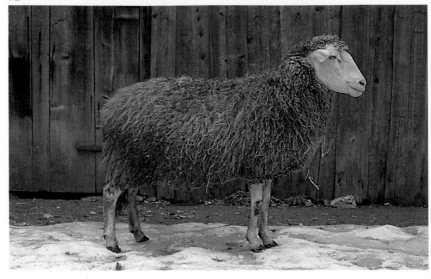

Forest

Characteristics: Small to medium-sized. Head slightly compressed and relatively short. Ears project horizontally from head. Fine limbs. Hard hooves. Close-wool. Mainly white, but there are light and dark brown animals. Polled.

	Ram	Ewe
Height at shoulder	65–70	60–65
Weight	60–70	45–50

Distribution: Bavarian Forest.
Uses: Placid, robust and hardy in bad weather. Aseasonal rutting. Lambs twice yearly, or at least three times in two years. Lambing percentage about 180%. Moderate capacity for fattening. Suitable for all-purpose crossing with meat-sheep breeds. Annual fleece yield 3.0 kg (ewes), 3.5 kg (rams).
Breed history: Old indigenous breed of the Bavarian Forest. Apparently originated in the Zaupel sheep, from which it was developed by crossing with other land races. As the original type was largely resistant to footrot, selection was performed for this characteristic after cross-breeding. The appearance was scarcely altered by this over the course of time. At the turn of the century, the Forest is thought still to have been predominantly horned. Several centuries ago, similar sheep occurred in the German Alpine regions and in the Mühlviertel in Austria. In 1976 the remaining animals were counted during a breeding experiment, when there were 248 ewes. The numbers are falling rapidly; there are now probably only 50 ewes on no more than four farms. The breed has also been designated the Bavarian Forest.

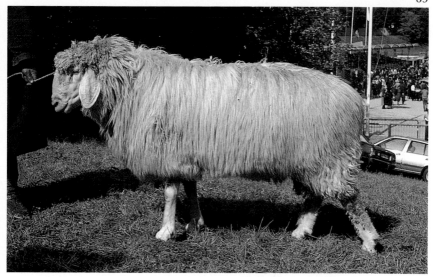

White Mountain

Characteristics: Medium build; long, white sheep with slightly compressed head and long, fleshy lop ears. Polled.

	Ram	Ewe
Height at shoulder	80–85	70–75
Weight	90–100	70–75

Distribution: Austrian Alps and foothills, the former Federal Republic of Germany, and Italy. Also isolated flocks outside this region.

Uses: Adapted to poor conditions and high precipitation. Hard hooves. Sure-footed, including on hills. Two fleeces per year. Annual fleece yield 4.5–5.5 kg (ewes), 6.5–7.5 kg (rams). Can mate at any time of year. First mating at 7–8 months. Lambing percentage 230%. Very good mothers.

Breed history: The Mountain goes back to the Zaupel or Stone and especially to the North Italian Bergamask. Originally there were many different strains, which were combined in Germany in the 1930s.

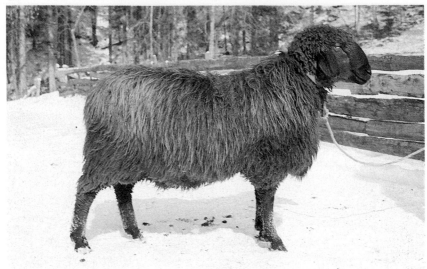

Brown Mountain

Characteristics: Medium-sized. Somewhat lighter than the white strain of Mountain. Wool light to rich brown. Head sharply compressed and narrow. Both sexes polled. Long, broad and fleshy lop ears. Closewool.

	Ram	Ewe
Height at shoulder	70–75	65–70
Weight	75–80	65–70

Distribution: German Alps and foothills, especially Tegernseer valley and Werdenfels region. Isolated holdings outside Bavaria, some even in north Germany. Similar animals in Austria and Italy, which would appear suitable for regenerating the stock.

Uses: Hardy. In summer usually graze high pastures. Adapted to harsh high-mountain climate. Like all mountain sheep, two fleeces per year. Annual fleece yield 6.0–7.0 kg (rams), 4.0–5.0 kg (ewes). Prolific. Lambing percentage 175%.

Breed history: In the past there were always occasional brown animals among the White Mountain. Duke Ludwig Wilhelm brought the first brown sheep from the Tyrol in 1934 and built up a flock of 100 animals before World War II. He required his hunters to have their uniforms made of his own brown wool. The small breed base eventually led to problems such as poor fertility and low bodyweight. It was believed that these characteristics could be improved by selective breeding, and in 1976 an application for recognition of the breed was made. In 1977, pre-flock-book development was started; the animals were given the current breed designation. The demand for undyed dark wool in recent years has meant that there are scarcely enough breeding animals now. About 20 flocks, but only five flock book enterprises; about 200 ewes.

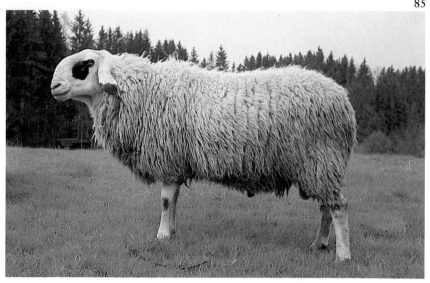

Carinthian Spectacled

Characteristics: Strong, medium-sized, long-legged sheep. Long head with very domed, narrow bridge of nose. Long, fleshy lop ears. White with black markings on the head, sometimes also on the body. When there is little pigmentation, the area in front of the eyes and the tips of the ears are black. When there is more pigmentation, the eyes have black rings and the outer two-thirds of the ears are also black. Sometimes there are black spots on the lips. The rest of the wool is white, and on the head it starts behind the ears. Closewool. Polled.

	Ram	*Ewe*
Height at shoulder	75–80	70–75
Weight	75–80	55–60

Distribution: South-east Bavaria. Summer grazing on Alpine pastures in Austria. Some animals live there all year.

Uses: Suited to mountain areas with annual precipitation of over 1000 mm. The close wool ensures that the rain does not penetrate the fleece. Hard hooves. Annual fleece yield 4.0–5.0 kg (ewes), 5.0–6.0 kg (rams). Lambing percentage 150%.

Breed history: Originated in Carinthia from crossing the old land sheep with the Bergamask and the related Paduan. Various names used in the past: Seeland, Bleiburg, Canaltal, Carinthian. Breed range extended over large parts of Austria, the Upper Bavarian Alps and the Alpine foothills of Bavaria. After 1938 almost completely displaced by standardisation of the Mountain sheep breeding target in Austria. Only a few remaining populations in the environs of Laufen (south-east Bavaria). The breed was given the current name there. It is also called the 'Carinthian Spiegel' or simply 'Carinthian'. Total population currently about 200 animals.

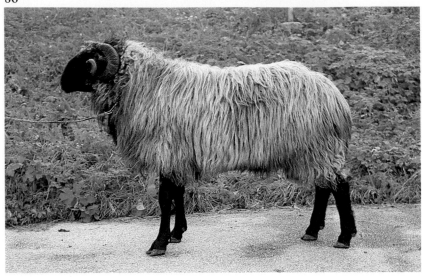

Tyrolean Stone

Characteristics: The animals may be pure white, grey with a black head and black legs, or pure black. Silky, shining, close wool with somewhat coarser outer fleece and finer inner fleece. Head compressed. Ears *do not* hang. Forehead wool-covered. Firm topline; strong constitution. Rams horned. Female animals hornless. The lambs of the grey and black types are always black.

	Ram	Ewe
Height at shoulder	80–85	70–80
Weight	80–100	70–85

Distribution: Tyrol. There are isolated flocks, sometimes crossed with other breeds, in other parts of Austria and in south Germany.

Uses: Suitable for mountainous regions, exceedingly sure-footed. Good fodder utilisation. Lean meat. High carcase yield. Two fleeces per year. Annual fleece yield 2.5–3.5 kg (ewes), 3.0–4.0 kg (rams). Very prolific, good rearing ability. Aseasonal rutting.

Breed history: Oldest Tyrolean sheep breed. Similar to extinct Zaupel. Was crossed with the Austrian and German Mountain and passed on to them its outstanding fertility. Immediately after the war there was a sharp drop in numbers. Since 1970 there has been a considerable increase, starting in the upper Ziller valley, owing to the efforts of interested breeders. A breed organisation was formed in 1974.

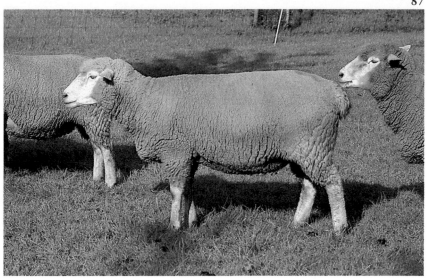

White Alpine

Characteristics: Broad body of medium length. Parts of body covered with wool and hair pure white. Occasionally there are small dark dots on the sides of the nose and on the ears. Broad, medium-length head with a wide muzzle. Bridge of the nose is straight. Ears are of medium length and extend horizontally. Haunches have broad, well-developed muscles extending well down. Polled.

	Ram	Ewe
Height at shoulder	74–78	67–73
Weight	80–100	60–80

Distribution: Most common sheep breed in Switzerland. Mainly eastern Switzerland, Tessin, the interior of Switzerland and the lower Valais.

Uses: Resistant to disease and severe weather. Suitable for mountain regions. Make modest demands on fodder and husbandry conditions. Meat. Annual fleece yield 3.5–4.5 kg (ewes). Good mothers, prolific milk yield. Generally, three lambings in two years. Mature moderately early.

Breed history: Eastern Switzerland, the interior of Switzerland and Tessin imported mainly Württemberg rams from 1929, and western Switzerland and the canton of Bern imported Ile de France animals from 1936. The breeds were resolved in 1938. Nevertheless, the designations 'White Alpine' (western Switzerland) and 'White Thoroughbred' or 'White' (elsewhere in Switzerland) continued to be used. Since 1978 the designation 'White Alpine' has been used for all pure white sheep in Switzerland.

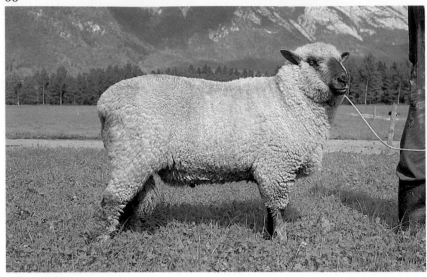

Brown-headed Mutton

Characteristics: Large build and strong constitution. Wool white. Body parts covered with hair (head, legs) are brown to black/brown. Polled.

	Ram	*Ewe*
Height at shoulder	72–78	68–74
Weight	80	70

Distribution: Switzerland.
Uses: Meat. Annual fleece yield 4.0–5.0 kg (ewes), 4.5–5.5 kg (rams). Lambing average is 1.6. As a rule lambs once a year, rarely twice.

Breed history: From 1870 English breeds (Suffolk, Southdown, Shropshire, Oxford Down) were imported into Switzerland and crossed with indigenous breeds. The Brown-headed Mutton existed at the end of the nineteenth century. At the start of the twentieth century, the German Black-headed Mutton was used for cross-breeding.

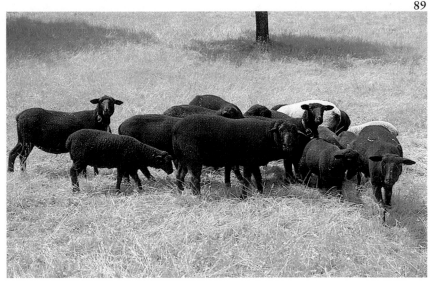

Black-brown Mountain

Characteristics: Medium-sized, deep and broad. Wool uniformly light brown through chestnut to black. Some wool on forehead. Body parts covered with hair (head and legs) are shiny black. In ewes the head is of medium length, in rams it is short; slightly compressed nose. Ears are of medium length and extend horizontally. Robust build. Good bone formation. Wide-set limbs. Polled.

	Ram	Ewe
Height at shoulder	73–78	66–72
Weight	70–90	60–65

Distribution: Switzerland. Mainly the cantons of Freiburg, Bern, Jura, Lucerne and Zürich. Isolated flocks outside Switzerland.
Uses: Healthy, strong constitution. Resistant to weather and diseases.

Suitable for mountainous regions. Make modest demands on fodder and husbandry conditions. Meat. Annual fleece yield 3.0–3.5 kg (ewes), 3.5–4.0 kg (rams). Ready to breed at the age of 8–10 months. As a rule, two lambings per year. Lambing average 1.7.
Breed history: Goes back on the one side to the Frutig (Frutigen in the Bernese Oberland), and on the other to the Jura. The former were crossed at the start of the nineteenth century with 'Flemish sheep' from the Netherlands and Belgium, and in the middle of that century with Spanish Merinos. The Jura was mostly brown and black at the end of the nineteenth century. At the start of the twentieth century, a black strain was bred from it. In other parts of Switzerland, lighter individuals – brown to golden – sometimes called Elb, were treated as an independent breed.

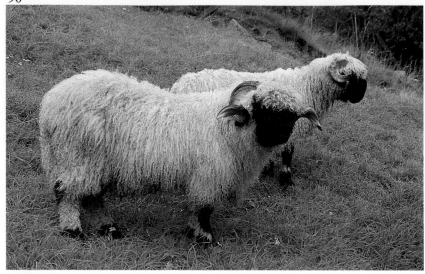

Valais Black-nosed

Characteristics: Large build, coarse wool. Wool uniformly white. Nose to centre of head and ears deep black. Eyes black-ringed. Legs black from pastern joint down. Black spots on hocks and front knees. Tail long and wool-covered. Nose very compressed. Horned. Horns corkscrew-shaped and extending to the sides of the head.

	Ram	Ewe
Height at shoulder	75–82	70–76
Weight	80–100	65–85

Distribution: Local breed of Upper Valais in Switzerland. Only found occasionally in other cantons. Isolated animals in the former West Germany.

Uses: Late-maturing land race, well suited to the harsh conditions in the mountains. It can utilise the steepest and stoniest meadows and is very loath to wander; it therefore does not need to be tended continuously. Meat. Annual fleece yield 3.0–4.0 kg (ewes), 3.5–4.5 kg (rams). Staple depth at 180 days 7–8 cm. Lambing percentage 140%.

Breed history: Goes back essentially to the Visper (valley) sheep, which was similar in appearance and was also horned. Although the term 'black-nosed breed' was first used in 1884, the breed has existed since at least the fifteenth century. About 1877 Cotswold rams from England and Germany were introduced into western Switzerland, and were apparently crossed with the ancestors of the Black-nosed. There may have been occasional cross-breeding with Bergamasks. When the breeds were resolved in Switzerland in 1938, no breed standard was established and no breeding target was set; this was not resolved until 1962. Two years later, the Black-nosed sheep was included in the Swiss Sheep Breed Society.

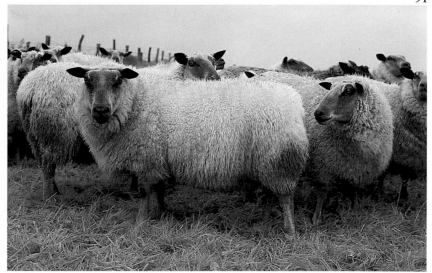

Blue-headed Mutton, Bleu de Maine

Characteristics: Large breed, white wool. There is no wool on the head to behind the ears or on the legs. The head and legs are slate-blue to blue-grey. Mucous membranes are black. The head seems broad and flat, but narrow at the muzzle. Prominent eyes. High-set, narrow, upright ears. The body is long, broad and deep. Pronounced haunches extend well down. Relatively fine limbs. Polled.

	Ram	Ewe
Height at shoulder	85–90	80–85
Weight	110–130	80–90

Distribution: France, the former Federal Republic of Germany (mainly North Rhine/Westphalia).
Uses: Suited to living in enclosures. Hardy. A real meat sheep. Lambs have good-quality carcases. High carcase yield. Annual fleece yield 4.0–4.5 kg (ewes), 5.0–6.0 kg (rams). Good milk production ensures that the lambs grow fast. Mature early. Largely seasonal reproduction. Lambing percentage 150–200%. Easy lambers. Good mothers and sucklers.

Breed history: Developed by crossing unimproved Marsh sheep with English meat sheep (Kent, Wensleydale), but narrower in the muzzle. In the former West Germany they have also been subjected to selective breeding since the start of the 1970s.

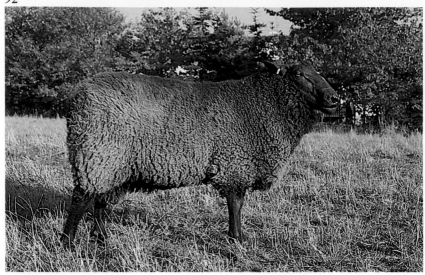

Black-Brown-Woolled Mutton

Characteristics: This designation covers the pure-bred pigmented versions of the Blue-headed Mutton (**91**) and the White–headed Mutton. The wool is initially black, but it bleaches considerably, especially in the summer, and the external visible part of the fleece becomes light brown. The lambs are born black. In shape and type these versions are the same as the relevant original breed.

Distribution: Rhineland.

Uses: Does not differ noticeably from the original breed. The wool is generally more ruffled and denser, so the fleece feels firmer. The hoped-for high demand for coloured wool and dark skins has not been entirely realised.

Breed history: Isolated pigmented animals occurred from time to time in the original breeds. In recent decades these have been deliberately collected by some breeders. Stock flocks have been formed in the Rhineland. The pigmented populations of both original breeds are kept in the same flock book, but they are not crossed.

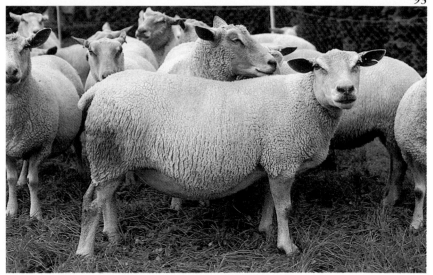

Charollais

Characteristics: Medium-sized to large. Parts covered in wool are white. The head has no wool; it often has spiky hairs, which can be pink to grey, and there are occasionally small black spots. Fine, long ears, the same colour as the head. Broad, flat forehead with widely set eyes. Long body with well-muscled back. Broad, deep brisket and adjoining shoulders. The wool is short and fine. Parts of legs without wool are brownish, quite short and powerful. Polled.

	Ram	Ewe
Height at shoulder	65	60
Weight	100–120	70–80

Distribution: France. The former Federal Republic of Germany (North-Rhine/Westphalia).
Uses: Good meat yield for both pure and crossbreeds. The lambs have daily weight gains of about 400 g. The carcase yield of rams is above 50%. Ewes have a high milk yield. Lambing percentage 180%.
Breed history: The breed developed at the beginning of the nineteenth century in the départements of Charollais, Morvan and Nivernais in central France. In 1825, English Dishley were crossed with them. Despite the introduction of other breeds (e.g. Southdown), the Charollais breed asserted itself in its original type after World War I. The Charollais sheep breed society was founded in 1963; 1,000 ewes in 24 flocks were entered in the flock book. By 1975 the population had risen to 6,800 registered animals. In 1974 the breed was officially recognised by the French agriculture ministry. There have been a few flocks in the former West Germany for some years.

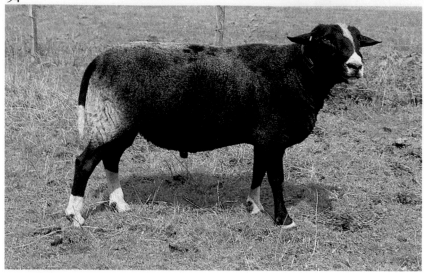

Zwartbles

Characteristics: Powerful, medium-sized, relatively short-legged sheep. Prick ears. Bridge of nose straight. Good depth and breadth to body. Well-developed udder. Tail of medium length. The basic colour is black/brown; old rams are occasionally greyish brown. White blaze, which starts behind the head and surrounds the muzzle but not the eyes. Occasionally the brisket is white. Legs white to a greater or lesser degree. Lower half of tail white. Tail wool-covered. Polled.

	Ram	Ewe
Height at shoulder	80–85	70–80
Weight	110–120	80–90

Distribution: Netherlands.
Uses: Undemanding. Prolific.
Breed history: The breed has been kept in the Netherlands for many decades. Appears to be similar to the Texel, but is probably related to the Milk sheep.

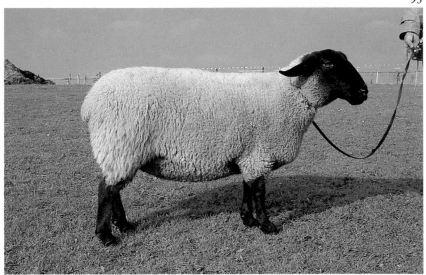

Suffolk

Characteristics: Medium to large. Wool white. Head and legs from front knee and tarsal joint down black. Unlike the Black-headed Mutton, the head has no wool to behind the ears. Bridge of nose slightly domed. Fairly large muzzle. Ears long, thin and somewhat drooping. Broad brisket extending well forwards. Long, broad back. Well-muscled haunches. Legs rather short. Polled.

	Ram	Ewe
Height at shoulder	70–80	60–70
Weight	100–120	70–85

Distribution: Originally UK; now also France, central Europe, New Zealand, Australia, and North and South America.
Uses: Demanding feeder. Suitable for enclosed and free-range husbandry. Outstanding meat formation. The meat is tender and lean. The lambs grow fast. Annual fleece yield 3.0–4.0 kg (ewes). Mature very early. Lambing percentage on average 140%. First mating possible in first year.
Breed history: The breed has been known since the end of the eighteenth century. It was developed by selection from cross-breeds of Norfolk with Southdown. It was initially known as Southdown-Norfolk and Blackface. Only when a special class was provided in 1859 at agricultural society shows in Suffolk did it receive its present name. In France and North America it is bred more extensively than the original British form. Often used to improve black-headed breeds. Kept in the former West Germany since the 1970s.

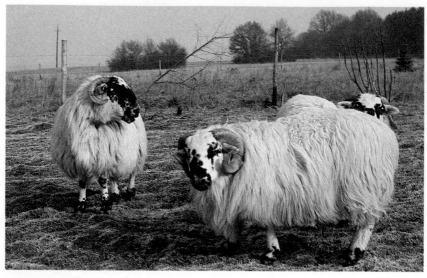

Scottish Blackface

Characteristics: Medium-sized. Mixed-wool. Strong bone formation. Broad head. Compressed nose. Long body. Broad pelvis. Back and haunches well muscled. Wool white. Head and legs white with black spots (black may predominate). Horned.

	Ram	Ewe
Height at shoulder	70	65
Weight	70–80	50–55

Distribution: The hilly areas of the UK, especially Scotland. Small numbers in other countries. Some animals in the former Federal Republic of Germany (Hunsrück).

Uses: Hardy. Contented. Adaptable. Resistant to the effects of bad weather. Tender meat. Annual fleece yield 3.5–4.0 kg. Wool fairly coarse. Mature late. Moderately prolific. Good milk yield. Much sought-after breed for cross-breeding.

Breed history: Belongs to the hill breeds of the UK. The Scottish Blackface is the most important branch of the old spotted British sheep. In the middle of the last century it was crossed with the Heath in north Germany.

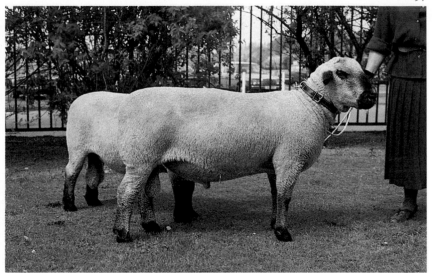

Hampshire

Characteristics: Large. Powerful build. Medium-length, broad head with prominent cheek bones. Ears are carried horizontally. Compressed nose. Deep body. Deep, domed brisket. Broad, fleshy back. Full haunches extending well down. Legs short. The white wool covers the cheeks and the upper part of the bridge of the nose. Front of legs bear wool down to the hooves. Parts of body covered with hair are dark brown to black. In the UK it is one of the short-wool meat sheep breeds.

	Ram	Ewe
Height at shoulder	85	80
Weight	100–140	70–90

Distribution: Mainly UK, where it is indigenous. North and South America, Australia, former USSR. Significant breed in France.

Uses: Robust. Matures early. Adaptable. Lambing percentage 155%. Good mothers. High milk yield. Lambs grow fast; average daily weight gains from tenth to thirtieth day after birth are 300 g for single lambs and 250 g for twin lambs; 25 kg at 70 days old. Generally not too fat. High carcase yield; top-quality meat. Well suited to crossing with other breeds for producing lambs for slaughter. Good fodder utilisation. Annual fleece yield about 4 kg.

Breed history: Developed selectively at the beginning of the nineteenth century in the south of England, especially Hampshire. About the middle of that century the breed was considerably modified by the breeder Mr Humphrey. For a while it was the best meat breed, very similar to the Oxfordshire breed. Introduced into France from the end of the nineteenth century. Imported into Germany at the start of this century, where it was crossed with the Black-headed Mutton.

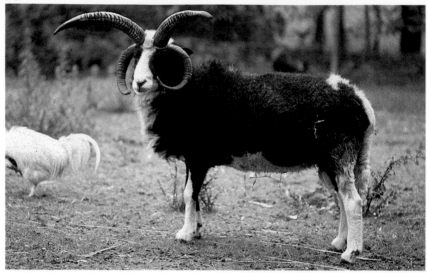

Jacob

Characteristics: Slim, medium-sized sheep. Animals with four or even six horns are particularly striking, although there are individuals with two horns or even none. The colours are black or brown with white. As a rule there are patches of colour, but there are also animals that are completely coloured with a few white markings, and almost completely white ones.

	Ram	Ewe
Height at shoulder	75–80	70–75
Weight	75–90	45–60

Distribution: UK. Have been kept in zoological gardens in Europe for many centuries. Recently favoured by private sheep farmers mainly because of the unusual wool. There is an extensive flock in Lower Rhine.
Uses: Robust. Contented. Wool prized owing to its colour. Fleece weight 2–3 kg.

Prolific. Lambing percentage 130–180%. Well-developed mothering characteristics. Birth weight about 3.6 kg.
Breed history: The breed was developed from a flock kept in a park in England in the eighteenth century. Subsequently, Jacobs were kept initially for ornamental reasons in parks and on farms. In 1969 a breed society was formed. By 1975 there were more than 150 registered flocks with a total of more than 3,000 animals. Today the population numbers many thousand. There are currently two different breeding aims: some breeders just want an extravagant sheep, whose usefulness is of secondary importance; other owners are trying, with some success, to increase bodyweight and prolificacy.

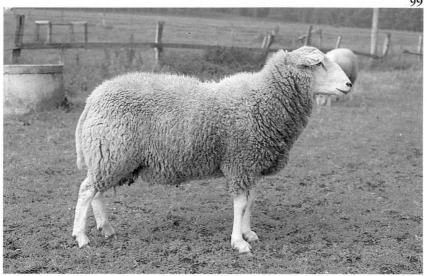

Flemish

Characteristics: As a rule completely white. In some animals the muzzle, nose and ears have spots of pigment. Head covered with hair to behind the ears. Short tail, sometimes covered with hair, sometimes with short wool. Similar to Texel, but with less muscle.

	Ram	Ewe
Height at shoulder	75–80	70–75
Weight	90–110	60–80

Distribution: Belgium, Netherlands. Some flocks in north Germany.

Uses: Very prolific; yearlings usually produce twins, mothers of three years or older produce on average three lambs. Used in cross-breeding programmes because of high fertility.

Breed history: Arose from Marsh sheep of coastal regions. In the nineteenth century, Texel, Milk and English Lincolns were crossed with them. Investigations of blood groups have shown that this breed is closer to the Texel than the Friesian Milk, its appearance being intermediate between the two. In the former West Germany it has been crossed with the Leine.

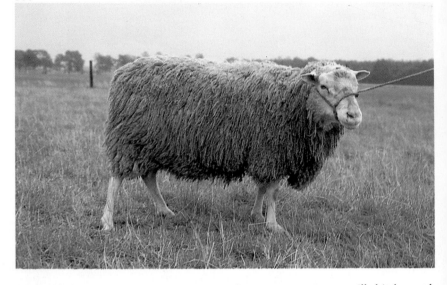

Finnish

Characteristics: Medium-sized land race with a fine build. Predominantly pure white, although there are occasional black, grey and brown animals. Head has no wool to behind the ears. Broad forehead. Small prick ears. The body is deep and long. Short tail. Mostly polled; occasionally there are horned rams.

	Ram	Ewe
Height at shoulder	70–75	65–70
Weight	80–90	60–70

Distribution: Finland. In recent decades it has been imported into many other countries with large-scale sheep rearing.
Uses: Undemanding. Hardy. Meat fullness corresponds to that of other land races. Annual fleece yield 2.5–4.0 kg (rams), 2.0–3.0 kg (ewes). Usually two fleeces per year. Most ewes lamb for the first time at one year old. Unusually high fertility of 200–400%; however, there are numerous still births and losses of lambs.

Breed history: Old land race of Finland and only sheep breed of this country which has considerable commercial significance. About 1960 there was for a time a considerable decline in the population in Finland, until international demand grew. Owing to its high prolificacy it has been crossed with many other sheep breeds for several decades and has also been kept as a pure breed outside Finland.

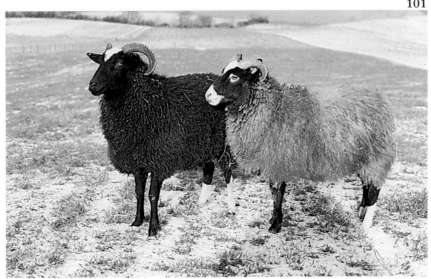

Gotland

Characteristics: Small to medium-sized sheep. Silver grey to dark brown. White markings on the head and legs. Close-wool. Short tail covered with hair. The animals of the original type have horns (**101**), while those bred now are mostly polled.

	Ram	Ewe
Height at shoulder	65	60
Weight	60–70	45–50

Distribution: Sweden, Denmark, the former East Germany. Some examples in north Germany.

Uses: Contented, robust and resistant to harsh weather. Undemanding with regard to fodder and husbandry. The annual fleece yield is about 4.0–6.0 kg. Two fleeces per year are necessary. Used for skins. Lambs are slaughtered at 4–5 months at a weight of 30–33 kg. Mature early; ready to breed at six months old. Older ewes produce 2 or 3 lambs, which they can easily rear as they produce a lot of milk.

Breed history: Oldest Swedish sheep breed. A small remnant of this breed has survived free of improvement on the island of Lilla Karlsö off the coast of Gotland. This population now numbers about 1,000 animals. In the former East Germany, animals are kept which have been modified by crossing with high–yield breeds. They are bred selectively for fast growth, wool yield, a contented nature, hardiness and suitability for keeping in isolation. Often mated with Milk sheep and subsequently used for displacement crossing with Gotland rams.

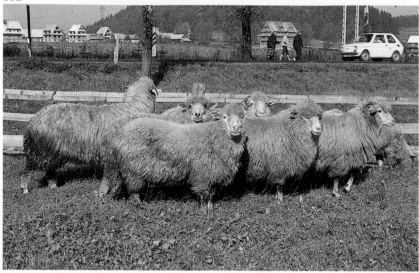

Cakiel, Polish Mountain

Characteristics: Small–framed. The wool is generally white; there are however also brown, black and spotted animals (which may not be entered in the flock book). Mixed–wool. Rams always horned, ewes sometimes.

	Ram	Ewe
Height at shoulder	55	50
Weight	55	40

Distribution: Podhale region at the foot of the High Tatra in southern Poland. In summer, found in other areas of southern Poland as well, because of a ban on grazing in the Tatra National Park.

Uses: Hardy. Undemanding. Suitable for free-range husbandry. The ewes are milked. The milk, about 70 kg in 5 months (fat content of 7%), is mainly made into a strong cheese. The fleece yield is 4 kg. The ratio of finer to coarser wool is about 1:2. Skins. Matures late. Lambing percentage is about 115%.

Breed history: Sheep breeding has been very important in Podhale for centuries. The animals originate in the free-range flocks of Zackel sheep of Walachian shepherds who came from Romania. After World War I, Pomeranian and Siebenburg Zackel sheep were crossed with them, and the East Friesian Milk was used to increase milk yield. After World War II, it was decided to unify the different strains and, in addition, Kent, Leicester and Leine, as well as Zigaya from Czechoslovakia, were crossed with them. The breed has become similar to the original mixed-wool type, although its weight has increased. The total population is now about 160,000 animals. The breed is mainly kept by farmers. Breeding in Germany, in which two government enterprises take part, is based on about 3,000 flock book ewes.

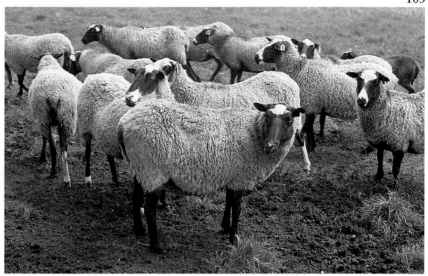

Romanov

Characteristics: Relatively small-framed. Mixture of black and white hairs gives various shades of greyish blue. The rams have a mane on the neck and back. White markings on head and legs. Closewool. Small head. Short tail without wool. Rams mostly horned; ewes hornless.

	Ram	Ewe
Height at shoulder	69	66
Weight	60–80	45–55

Distribution: Originally former Soviet Union. Now also numerous other countries; mainly France, but also the former West Germany.

Uses: Undemanding and hardy. They withstand cold and great temperature fluctuations. Good milk yield. Good furs from older lambs; the skins of adult animals are also prized as furs. Annual fleece yield is 3–4 kg (rams), 2–3 kg (ewes). In the former Soviet Union they generally have three fleeces per year. Aseasonal. Exceedingly prolific; the ewes produce 2–4, and occasionally 5 lambs. Are now crossed with some other breeds to improve their fertility.

Breed history: Derives originally from the Tutayev region on the Volga (former Soviet Union). This breed is traced back to the northern Short-tailed sheep. It was developed towards the end of the seventeenth century from indigenous breeds by selecting animals for fertility and skin quality.

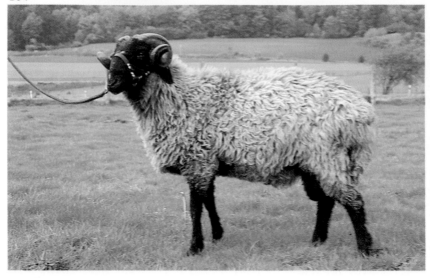

Karakul

Characteristics: Lean Steppe sheep of medium size. The coloration ranges from dirty brown through light to dark grey and blue/grey to black/brown shades. The legs from the front knee and tarsal joint up are black. The lambs are born black, grey, brown, golden or pink. Longish, narrow head with somewhat compressed nose. Generally have broad, long flop ears. Belong to the fattailed sheep, i.e. they store as much as several kg of fat in the subcutaneous tissue of the upper part of the tail. Rams horned. Ewes hornless or with horn stumps.

	Ram	Ewe
Height at shoulder	70	65
Weight	60–70	40–50

Distribution: Former Soviet Union, former GDR, Afghanistan, Namibia, South America and the USA. In many other countries there are only a few animals.

Uses: Undemanding, hardy, long-lived. Adapted to dry steppe and semi-desert regions. Most important fur sheep breed in the world. The skins of lambs slaughtered at a few days old give Persian Lamb. Mixed-wool. The wool is used for weaving and carpet making. Annual fleece yield 2.0 kg (ewes), 3.3 kg (rams). The meat has a game-like flavour. Seasonal reproduction. As a rule there is only one lamb.

Breed history: Originated in west Turkistan, where it had been bred for at least 900 years. In the second half of the nineteenth century and at the start of this century, Karakuls were taken to other parts of the Soviet Union. They arrived in Afghanistan in 1877. At the start of this century the breed was built up in Namibia, from where it has been exported to many other countries. Karakuls are sometimes crossed with Heath and other breeds of the German-speaking countries.

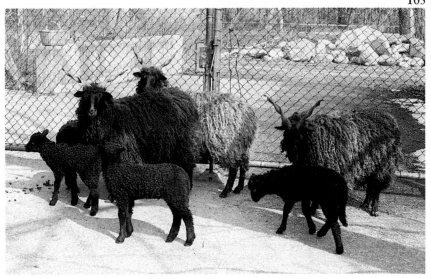

Hungarian Zackel, Racka

Characteristics: Small and dainty. Mixed-wool. Long shaggy fleece. Narrow head. Forehead and tail wool-covered. There are two types: white and grey. The lambs of the white Zackels are born light-golden to dark brown; the lambs of the grey strain have a black, ruffled skin that resembles that of Karakuls. Horned. The very long horns of old animals are elongated and twisted like a corkscrew. They form a V-shape.

	Ram	Ewe
Height at shoulder	60	55
Weight	60–70	40–45

Distribution: Hungary, especially the Debrecen region. Small populations in neighbouring countries. There are other Zackel sheep breeds from Turkey to the Carpathians.
Uses: Undemanding. Vigorous. Lively.

Prolific. Lambing percentage about 115%. Good milk yield, so they are sometimes milked. During a lactation period of 100 days they give up to 70 kg of milk. Tasty meat. Annual fleece yield 2.0–3.0 kg. Skins originally used for clothing by the shepherds.
Breed history: It is generally assumed that the Hungarians brought this breed with them when they migrated to their present location about 1,100 years ago. Earlier it was widely dispersed. Because of its original appearance and the unusual horns it is often kept in animal parks. It is increasingly prized by private sheep farmers. Gene reserves are kept in the Puszta area and in the National Park of Hortobagy. A breed society, together with government institutions, is engaged in preserving the breed. The total population is about 4,500 animals.

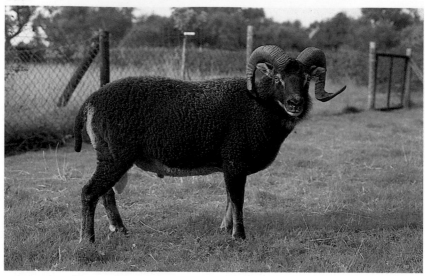

Soay

Characteristics: Small sheep with very short, dense wool that does not need to be shorn. (The wool grows about 7 cm per year.) Short, hair-covered tail. Rams have an incipient neck mane. Occasionally light brown or grey, but mostly dark brown; the belly, backs of thighs and legs, the area around the eyes and the insides of the ears are pale. After moulting in June, the wool is dark, but it becomes lighter during the summer. The rams and about half the ewes have horns.

	Ram	Ewe
Height at shoulder	50–55	45
Weight	26–30	20–25

Distribution: Various islands off the coast of Scotland as well as (animal) parks in the UK. For some years there have also been some on the European mainland. The former Federal Republic of Germany, mainly in Rhineland-Palatinate.

Uses: Robust and undemanding. Suitable for landscape maintenance. Produce 0.5–1.5 kg wool, but the fleece is unconventional. Temperamental; behave like wild animals. Cannot be driven by dogs. Lambing percentage 130%

Breed history: The breed originates on the island of Soay, one of the St. Kilda islands in the north-west of Scotland. The animals lived there largely independently. Comparisons of skeletons show that they do not differ from the domesticated sheep of the Neolithic Age and the Bronze Age. According to old reports, there were about 500 sheep on Soay in 1698. In 1931 the Marquis of Bute bought the uninhabited group of islands. In 1932 he brought 107 sheep from Soay to Hirta, the largest island of the group, to increase the population. There are now several thousand animals.

Goats

The word Ziege (goat) is derived from the Germanic 'tig' or 'tik', which means 'small domestic animal'. Presumably the meaning was more general previously, namely 'small animal'.

This can still be seen in the English 'tick'. In German, too, the words 'Ziege' and 'Zecke' (tick) are very similar.

Goats occur all over the world except near the poles. There are about 450 million in all; their number is growing. This applies especially to semi-arid and arid regions, where it is scarcely possible to keep other domestic animals. They are also numerous in areas where certain species of animal (cattle, pigs) may not be killed or eaten.

Goats can be very undemanding. If there is no other feed available they will eat kitchen scraps or even paper. This does not mean that they are not fond of nibbling or that they do not deliberately and carefully select the tastiest morsels from a wider range of feed. Goats can jump and climb very well. It is difficult to make fences high and secure enough to contain them. As they like to eat foliage, they can cause considerable damage in gardens and, in the long term, in forests. The karst landscape of the fringes of the Mediterranean and its islands and of other regions is traced back to goat-keeping. This disadvantge has caused some governments to ban goat-keeping totally or in certain areas. Today we know that this view is not entirely correct. With planned grazing and limited stocking densities, goats can be used in an ecological way. It is only unrestricted spreading of populations, mainly of feral goats, which makes ecological catastrophes unavoidable.

Goats are kept for milk, meat and skins, and some breeds also for wool. Good milk goats produce an annual milk yield corresponding to 20 times their bodyweight. It has not yet been possible to confirm experimentally that goat's milk does have the healing effect popularly attributed to it. However, it cannot be denied that goat's milk is a good substitute for cow's milk for those allergic to the latter. When collected in a clean manner, its taste is scarcely different from cow's milk. Goat's milk anaemia, feared in the past, is not due to the characteristics of the milk but to the overall nutritional situation of the people concerned. Zeus, the supreme god of the Ancient Greeks, is said to have been reared on goat's milk.

Kid's meat is a prized delicacy. Demand for it has risen in recent years in the German-speaking countries due to the increasing numbers of people from southern countries living there. As a result, a breed of meat goat, the Boer, is now kept in the former Federal Republic of Germany.

There are several breeds of goat whose wool is shorn and processed. The most important is the Angora, which came originally from Asia Minor, and which still has its largest population of two million animals in Turkey. The wool of this breed is sold as mohair. This word derives from the Arabic mukhayyar, which means 'best fleece'. It is difficult to keep the Angora goat in our temperate climate. It is very sensitive to the cold, especially after shearing. Another wool-producing breed is the Kashmir goat in central Asia, whose wool is sold under the same name. It produces the finest wool ever used in textiles. An individual hair has a diameter of less than $15\,\mu$m (for comparison: Merino wool has a diameter of about $25\,\mu$m).

A limiting factor in goat keeping is the strong smell, especially of the billies. Some goat-keeping enterprises have been abandoned because no one was willing to keep a billy. This dilemma can be partially resolved by artificial insemination. In the past, selective breeding in Germany was aimed at producing polled animals. If animals are polled, there is less danger of injury among the animals themselves and of harm to humans. Initially, however, the fact was overlooked that the polled factor is often associated with infertility among billies and the occurrence of hermaphrodites.

In the Middle Ages, goats were associated with devils and witches. The devil was often signified with a goat's foot. The reasons for the low regard in which goats were held were presumably the strong smell, their lively nature (the word 'capricious' is derived from the Latin for goat, capra, and describes their character), and the male's proverbially well-developed sexual instinct. Yet the goat has rendered outstanding service to man's welfare as no other animal. As the 'small man's cow', kept mostly in dark dungeons and fed on scraps, it helped people in towns to survive hard times. Other animal species kept in such conditions would have been unproductive and would not have produced young. The goat, however, remains trusting and friendly. It is not without reason that a German animal breeding official prefaced a book with the words 'the goat is the workers' sunshine' (Schaper, 1934).

Of approximately 200 breeds of goat in the world, only two are indigenous to the former German Federal Republic. Considerably more, namely eight, occur in Switzerland. Several reasons are put forward for this. However, it is remarkable that a country with a similar geographical position, namely Austria, has produced only one independent breed of goats. Of the approximately 40,000 goats kept in the former West Germany, 30% are White German Improved and 70% are Coloured German Improved.

The numbers of goats of individual breeds in Switzerland is shown in Table 11. Here, as in other central European countries, there has been a rapid decline in populations since World War II, which did not stop until the 1970s. In recent years the number of goats has remained stable.

Table 11. Numbers of goats in Switzerland by breed.

	1941	1961	1978 No.	%
Saanen	43,338	23,353	17,702	22.1
Appenzell	6,683	3,034	3,155	3.9
Toggenburg	20,082	8,869	8,635	10.8
Chamois-coloured Mountain	29,373	16,366	14,420	18.0
Bünden Striped	19,399	9,451	6,323	7.9
Verzasca	9,503	8,947	11,347	14.2
Valais Black-necked	7,656	2,166	2,972	3.7
Others	78,672	17,171	15,423	19.3
Total	214,706	89,357	79,977	100

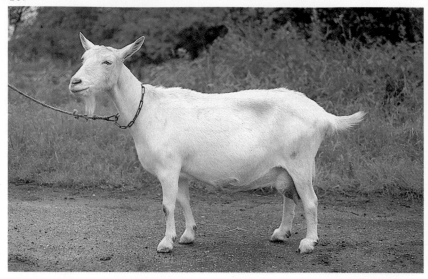

White German Improved

Characteristics: Powerfully built goat. Pure white. Sometimes slight reddish-yellow colouring on neck and back or flecks of pigment on nose, ears and udder. Coat is short and smooth. Males sometimes have longer hair on the neck and back. Polled.

	Male	Female
Height at shoulder	80–90	70–80
Weight	70–80	60–70

Distribution: Predominantly the northern half of the former Federal Republic of Germany as well as North Baden. The former German Democratic Republic.
Uses: Meat, skins. Annual milk yield 950 kg (3.5% fat). Highest yields are over 1800 kg. On average 2.1 kids per female per year.
Breed history: White goats have been known in central Europe for centuries. There have been pure white strains since the start of the nineteenth century (e.g. Langensalza), which were eventually incorporated into the White German Improved. The milk yield was already prized at that time. From 1880 the Saanen and the Appenzell were crossed with the white German goat strains and sometimes kept as pure breeds. In 1928 all white goats were brought into one breed and have since been known by the present name. After World War II, the number of animals fell continuously until a few years ago when the situation levelled off or even improved slightly.

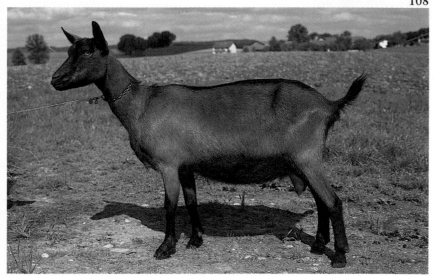

Coloured German Improved

Characteristics: Coat short and smooth. Mainly polled. Three colourings:

- *Dark brown base colour.* Black back line. Underbelly and legs from hock and front knee down are black (earlier Franconian).
- *Medium- to rich-brown base colour.* Dark brown or black back line. Underbelly light brown. Legs from the hock and front knee down have a dark brown sheen. Suggestion of a light stripe from the base of the horn to the corner of the muzzle (earlier Black Forest).
- *Light greyish brown.* Underbelly and legs from hock and front knee down are ochre. Light stripe from above the eye to the corner of the muzzle (Thuringian Forest, earlier German Toggenburg).

Distribution: Predominantly southern Germany, in the former GDR.

Uses: Meat. Skins. Annual milk yield 900 kg (3.7% fat). Highest yield of 1,800 kg. Young: 2.1 kids per female per year. First mating possible at seven months.

	Male	Female
Height at shoulder	75–85	70–80
Weight	60–80	50–65

Breed history: Until the end of the nineteenth century there were brown goats in addition to other colour strains in all regions of Germany. Only at the beginning of this century were goats of uniform coloration and type kept, often only in small areas. In 1928, the Imperial Association of German Goat Breed Societies decided that all coloured strains would be combined under the designation 'Coloured German Improved', to maintain a larger breeding base.

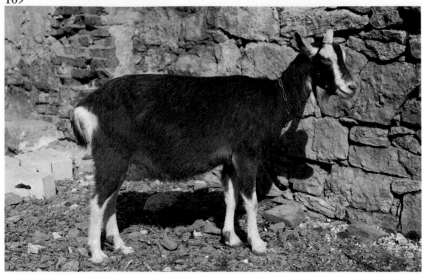

Thuringian Forest

Characteristics: Medium-sized and powerfully built. Coat short and smooth. Males are generally 'trousered', i.e. they have long hair on the rump and upper thighs. Chocolate brown with no foxy sheen and no back line. Distinctive face mask: white band from the area above the eye to the upper lip. There is a white line around the ears and muzzle. The 'escutcheon' under the tail is white. The belly is dark. The lower legs are white. Prick ears. Slender neck. Brisket deep and broad with well-sprung ribs. Straight, long back. Moderately sloping rump. Powerful and well-muscled limbs. Well-developed udder.

	Male	Female
Height at shoulder	80–85	70–75
Weight	65–75	50–60

Distribution: South-eastern area of the former GDR. There are animals of a similar type in northern Bavaria in the former Federal Republic of Germany.

Uses: Hardy and undemanding. Meat. Skins. Annual milk yield (at least 180 days) is about 1,000 kg (3.9% fat).

Breed history: Goats were introduced from Switzerland to improve goat breeding in Thuringia. Towards the end of the century, Toggenburgs were introduced. Crossing the 'Thuringian Toggenburgs' with the indigenous goats by selective breeding produced a uniform type, renamed the 'Thuringian Forest' in 1935 and subsequently admitted to shows. After a short period of success post-war, populations declined sharply in subsequent decades. The animals have become smaller and lighter. The population of animals of the Thuringian Forest type in the former GDR is estimated to be 1000. Only some of these are pure-bred, however. Breeder organisations are devoted to preserving this endangered breed.

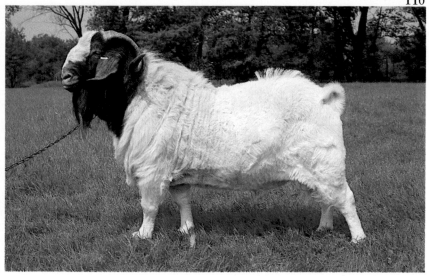

Boer, Meat

Characteristics: Large, long-legged goat. White with a reddish-brown head and neck. White blaze. Body sometimes has brown patches. Powerful head with compressed nose. Broad, fleshy withers. Well-developed broad brisket and well-sprung ribs. Broad back. Muscular legs. Overall appearance is powerful. Short, soft hair. Long lop ears. Horned.

	Male	Female
Height at shoulder	82–90	65–80
Weight	80–90	50–70

Distribution: South Africa, Namibia, East Africa, the former West Germany.
Uses: Very good meat development. Kids have high daily weight gains. Wethers achieve a weight of up to 100 kg without concentrates. Carcase yield about 50%. Tasty, tender meat, which does not have the characteristic goat odour. The skins are made into shoes, gloves and book covers. Very prolific. Good mothers.

Breed history: Native to South Africa. It is derived from the Hottentot goat, which in turn is traced back to imported Nubian goats. It may have been crossed with goats from Europe and India. The original form is thought to have been small and spotted. Since the start of this century, selective breeding has been performed for meat formation. There has been a flock book since 1959. The first Boers were brought to Germany several years ago for the purpose of developing meat goat breeding to meet the increased demand for kid meat. As there are only a few Boer goats, developing a meat goat population in the former Federal Republic of Germany requires displacement crossing with indigenous breeds.

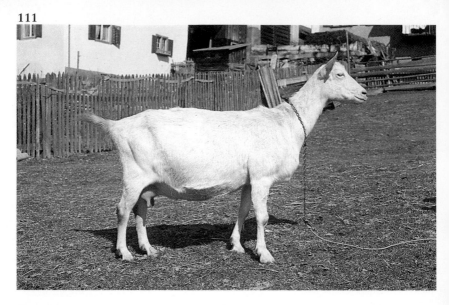

Saanen

Characteristics: Pure white, short-haired. There are often spots of pigment over the whole body, but only on the skin, not the hair. They can also be seen on parts of the body with sparse hair, such as the head and udder. Mostly polled; however, in recent years, increasingly horned.

	Male	Female
Height at shoulder	80–95	75–85
Weight	75	50

Distribution: Western half and north of Switzerland. There is scarcely a country where goats are kept for milk, which has not imported Saanen goats. In 14 European countries there is a breed that is called 'Saanen'.

Uses: Meat. Skins. The average annual milk yield in Switzerland is 750kg; this yield is all the more remarkable in that it is generally achieved with the farm's own fodder and without great addition of concentrates. Highest yields about 3500kg.

Breed history: It was bred in the nineteenth century for white coloration, short hair and the polled factor. It was already regarded as a good milker and hence was imported by numerous countries, where it was sometimes kept as a pure breed and kept its original name. It originates in the Saanen region and Upper Simmental (canton of Bern). From here it spread initially across parts of central Switzerland. In 1890 breeders formed a breed cooperative in order to conduct planned breeding and exportation. Best known and for a long time the most successful goat breed in the world.

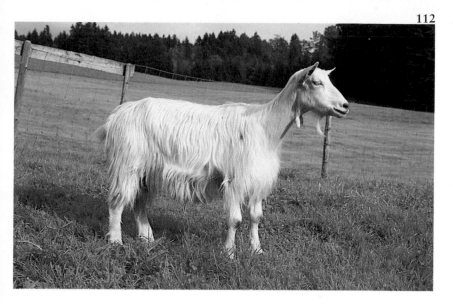

Appenzell

Characteristics: White, sometimes with a hint of pink. The hair is long, especially on the croup and upper thighs. Originally hornless, now increasingly horned.

	Male	Female
Height at shoulder	70–80	65–70
Weight	65	45–50

Distribution: North-east Switzerland, especially the two Appenzell cantons. North America. UK. Small numbers in the former West Germany.

Uses: Meat. Skins. Average annual milk yield 680 kg. This represents a considerable increase in yield since 1962–63 (408 kg).

Breed history: In the Appenzell cantons at the end of the last century, goats were bred which were black, reddish or spotted as well as being short-haired. However, most animals of the 'Appenzell strain' were already white and long-haired. Such 'shaggy goats' were preferred, especially for summer grazing on high pastures. In 1903 a goat breeding cooperative was formed 'to preserve the white polled Appenzell goat as a pure breed and to improve it'. It should be emphasised that the 'white Appenzell goat' is quite different from the Saanen goat. Apart from having long hair, it is more stocky and has a shorter, broader head. In the nineteenth century it was already being exported to Germany in the form of the Saanen goat, where it was crossed with the white strains. The Appenzell constitutes only 4% of the Swiss goat population; it is thus one of the least widely distributed breeds in that country. The number of flock book animals is almost 1000. The Appenzell is generally grouped with the Zürich goat, which is similar, although more like the Saanen.

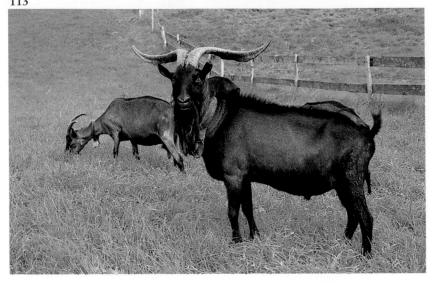

Chamois-coloured Mountain

Characteristics: Brown with a black underside, black legs from the hock and front knee down, a black back line, a black tail and black markings on the head. It occurs in two strains: the Oberhasli-Brienz type is polled, while the Graubünden (113) is horned.

	Male	*Female*
Height at shoulder	75–85	70–80
Weight	65	45

Distribution: Switzerland. The (originally) hornless type occurs in the Brienz region, in Greyerzerland and the rest of western Switzerland. The horned type occurs in the cantons of Graubünden and Uri. Similarly marked breeds of goat occur in many countries (e.g. Coloured German Improved, Pinzgau in Austria).
Uses: Meat, skins. The annual milk yield of the Oberhasli-Brienz type is 680 kg, and of the Graubünden type 570 kg. The latter is more robust, is kept in harsher conditions and withstands extreme climates.
Breed history: It can obviously be traced back to goats of an unnamed breed that corresponded to the current form in colour and markings and occurred in early Switzerland. These were, however, small and stocky and had a 'wild appearance' and were said to 'exhibit traces of the earliest stock of the early Swiss goat strain'. Later, a 'chamois-coloured Alpine breed' was mentioned, which consisted of several strains, at that time exclusively horned. The Oberhasli-Brienz type was bred for the polled factor in subsequent decades. Only in recent years has the trend towards horned animals returned. The Chamois-coloured Mountain has been exported to many countries.

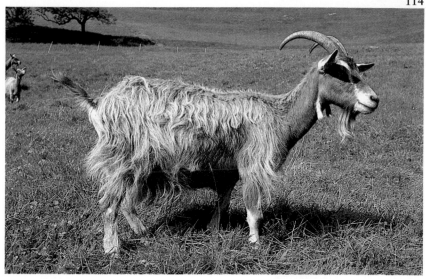

Toggenburg

Characteristics: Light brown to mousy grey with paler ears, paler stripes from the base of the ear to the muzzle and a white area around the muzzle. The legs from the hock and front knee down, as well as the rear of the thighs and the anus and vulva are also almost white. It is generally long-haired, primarily on the rear half of the body (coat), while the breeding trend is now towards short hair for hygiene reasons. In North America, this breed is exclusively short-haired. Polled and horned.

	Male	Female
Height at shoulder	75–85	70–80
Weight	65–75	45–50

Distribution: The canton of St. Gallen as well as central Switzerland. UK. North America. Isolated animals in southern Germany.

Uses: Meat, skins. Average annual milk yield 700–800 kg.

Breed history: Old local breed. Mentioned as early as 1802. Initially it occurred only in Toggenburg in the canton of St. Gallen in Switzerland, and then it slowly spread across its modern range and became prized internationally. At the start of this century it sometimes still had dark, or, increasingly, white spots or a completely dark coat, and was frequently horned. In central Europe it was occasionally crossed with other breeds in the past. At about the turn of the century it was exported to Germany where it was bred as an independent breed for some time. It represents 10.4% of the total Swiss goat population.

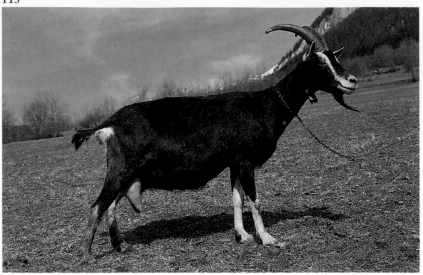

Bünden Striped

Characteristics: Anthracite to black. The following parts of the body are pale: ears, area around the muzzle and stripes from the base of the horns to the muzzle, underside of the tail, area around the anus, rear of the thigh (skirt), underbelly to the brisket, and legs from the hock and front knee down (boots). Short-haired. Horned.

	Male	Female
Height at shoulder	75–85	70–75
Weight	65	45–50

Distribution: Graubünden in Switzerland, UK.
Uses: Very hardy. Often covers great distances every day at a great altitude. The annual milk yield of on average 460 kg is considerable in these circumstances. Meat, skins.
Breed history: Mentioned in the literature at the start of the nineteenth century. At the beginning of the twentieth century described as the 'Black Bünden', when there were animals with the current markings as well as all-black animals. Recently the stock has been enhanced with animals of the same breed from the UK.

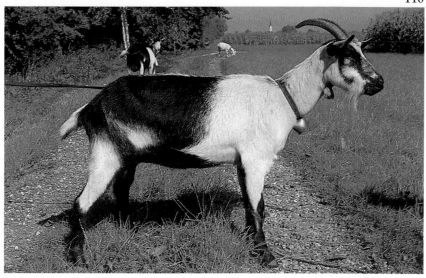

Peacock

Characteristics: The front half of the body is predominantly white with black 'boots', while the rear is predominantly black. However, the inside of the ears and the area around the muzzle are dark, and there are dark spots on the cheeks and dark stripes from the base of the horns over the eyes to the nose. These markings gave the breed its name. The upper side of the tail and the outside of the thigh is white; there is a white patch on the flank. Occasionally the whole coat has a brownish tinge. Dense, medium–length coat. Horned.

	Male	Female
Height at shoulder	75–85	65–75
Weight	70–80	50–60

Distribution: Graubünden and Ticino in Switzerland. Animals with similar coloration can be found in Austria, Upper Italy and in Haute Savoie. From there they went to North America as the French Alpine.

Uses: Meat, skins. The milk yield during the lactation of about seven months is on average 470 kg.

Breed history: Descriptions of the Prättigau and Engadine goat correspond largely with that of today's Peacock with regard to build, coat, horns and colouring. Once widely distributed in Graubünden and Ticino. After the reorganisation of goat breeds in Switzerland in 1938, when it was not officially recognised, the population declined sharply. It was maintained that it was a colour variant of the Bünden Striped, and that preserving it was not justified. Examinations of blood groups have revealed the Peacock to be closely related to this and to the Nera Verzasca. It does however seem to be distinctive and some breeders have continued to breed it for decades. Only about 300 animals exist.

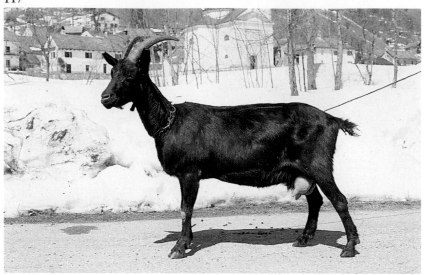

Nera Verzasca

Characteristics: Mostly completely black or black with a reddish–brown tinge on the thighs. Occasionally chocolate brown. Sometimes they have white markings and patches. Short–haired. Predominantly horned.

	Male	Female
Height at shoulder	80–90	75–85
Weight	70	50–55

Distribution: Ticino in Switzerland.
Uses: Hardiest goat breed in Switzerland. Adapted to extremely high and low temperatures. Very contented. Meat, skins. Annual milk yield 490 kg.
Breed history: Colour variants other than black occurred more frequently in the past, and in the current region of distribution there were shortand long–haired animals. This breed has always been undemanding and hardy. The breeding centre is the Verzasca valley, which extends from the northern end of Lago Maggiore northwards. Verzasca goats are kept in quite large numbers, particularly in the village of Sonogno at the end of the valley. The goats of several owners are sometimes housed in communal buildings. In the spring the goats range freely in the valley bottom.

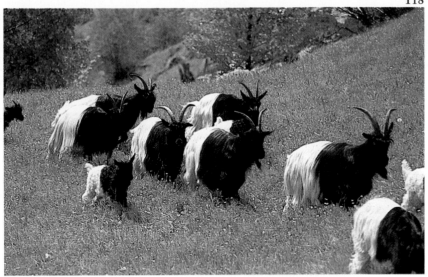

Valais Black-necked

Characteristics: Stocky high-mountain breed. Short head. Broad forehead and muzzle. Slightly protruding ears. Short neck. Straight back with broad loin. Muscular thighs. Front half of body black, rear half white. Long–haired. Horned.

	Male	Female
Height at shoulder	75–85	70–80
Weight	65–70	45–50

Distribution: Upper Valais in Switzerland. Mainly the Visp valleys, Zermatt and Saas Fee. In the former West Germany they are kept in numerous zoos, and occasionally in private animal collections. The Bagot goat in the UK has similar colouring.

Uses: A tourist attraction in the Valais. Remarkable fattening capability. Annual milk yield 580 kg.

Breed history: Originally mainly in the Lower Valais, then later also in the Upper Valais. According to historical reports it was introduced into this area by incoming African peoples in AD930. The 'glacier goat' was for a long time numerically the smallest of the recognised breeds in Switzerland. In 1974 the population had fallen to 440 animals. It has recovered somewhat in recent years. It constitutes 2.2% of the total Swiss goat population. In the past it was also called Saddle, Vispental and Halsene (French Race de Viège).

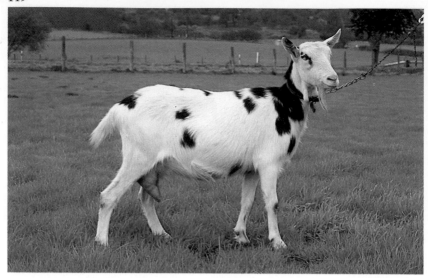

Dutch Spotted

Characteristics: Medium-sized. White with patches of black, grey or brown. Mostly short-haired. As a rule, the head and neck are extensively pigmented. Long body. Deep, broad brisket. Short pelvis. Relatively long–legged. Most animals are horned, but polled animals also occur.

	Male	Female
Height at shoulder	80–82	71–73
Weight	70	50–60

Distribution: Originally the Dutch provinces of South Holland and Zeeland. Now it occurs in other parts of the Netherlands and in Belgium, and there are some populations in northern Germany.

Uses: Undemanding. Hardy. Low susceptibility to disease. There are no data available on milk yield. Mature early. Prolific.

Breed history: It was developed in the Netherlands at the beginning of this century from land races subjected to little selective breeding, by crossing with Toggenburgs and Saanens from Switzerland and White Improved from Germany. Toggenburgs were crossed with it again in the 1940s. However, characteristics indicative of crossing with Toggenburgs are now undesirable. As a result of the efforts of the Dutch foundation for 'Rare Live-stock Breeds', the 'Dutch Organisation for Goat Breeding' opened a flock book in 1980. The number of registered animals is now about 800.

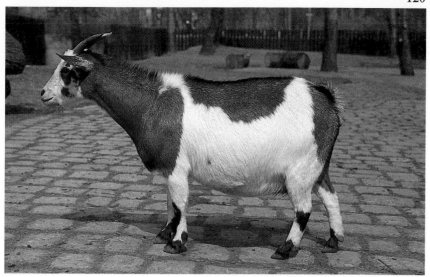

West African Dwarf

Characteristics: Achondroplastic dwarf with short legs, a short body and a large belly. It may be black, white, grey or brown. The animals generally have patches of colour. Short, broad head. Short prick ears. Horned.

	Male	Female
Height at shoulder	50	40–45
Weight	30	25

Distribution: West Africa. Now also Europe and North America. Other forms of dwarf goat occur in Central and East Africa as well as in India and Bangladesh.

Uses: Kept for meat and the skin in its countries of origin. The milk yield is low; hardly any is obtained. In Europe and North America it is kept in zoos, as a hobby, and as an experimental animal. Individuals are often kept in horse enterprises, to prevent the horses becoming bored.

Breed history: Mainly occurs in rain forest areas and on humid steppes, to which it is well suited. It is assumed to have come from Asia via Egypt. It was introduced to Europe many decades ago.

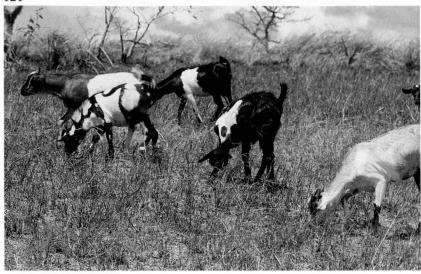

East African Dwarf

Characteristics: It does not have the short legs and large belly of the West African Dwarf, but is a well-proportioned breed with quite long legs. The animals look slim and elegant. The forehead line is straight or slightly indented. The ears are generally short and upright, but lop ears occur in some regions. The hair is short and soft. The colouring varies considerably: black, white, brown (sometimes with a black belly like the Franconian or with a pale belly like the Black Forest). Of the animals with patches of colour, those with white patches on a coloured background stand out (moon patches). Generally, both sexes have horns. The horns curve sharply backwards.

Distribution: Large areas of East Africa, except the hot, humid regions.
Uses: Undemanding and very adaptable. Suitable for utilising extreme locations. Although not heavily muscled, main use is for meat production. The milk is scarcely enough for the kid. Contributes essentially to providing protein for the poorer and thus cashless population and for people living in areas where other livestock species cannot be kept for ecological or economic reasons. Largely seasonal reproduction. As a rule there is only one kid (birth weight about 2 kg).
Breed history: Old land race. In provincial husbandry it has never been subjected to selective breeding. On test stations, East African Dwarf goats are sometimes crossed with European breeds or with the Boer goat to improve economic efficiency.

	Male	Female
Height at shoulder	65	60
Weight	30	25

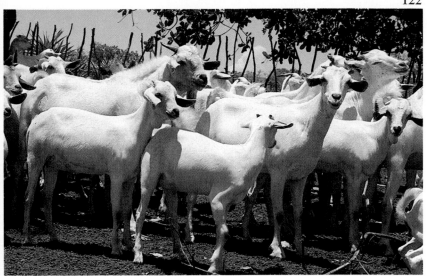

Galla, Somali

Characteristics: Slim, medium-sized goat. Uniform in conformation. Generally pure white. There is sometimes a reddish tinge, or black or brown spots on the ears and round the eyes. Rarely there is a black back line. The skin has black pigmentation, which is particularly noticeable on parts of the body with sparse hair or no hair. Short-haired. Relatively small head with concave nose line. Narrow, close-lying ears of medium size. Long neck. Long legs. Good muscling. Large, firmly attached udder. The males have a short beard; the females have no beard. The scrotum of the males is divided up to the body, so each testis has a separate scrotum. This seems to be an adaptation to high temperatures (cooling effect) or to awkward grazing conditions. Males are horned. The relatively short horns are turned outwards. Females often have only horn stumps or are hornless.

	Male	*Female*
Height at shoulder	70–75	65–70
Weight	35–55	30–45

Distribution: Somalia, the Ogaden province of Ethiopia, and north-east Kenya.

Uses: Undemanding. Adapted to high temperatures and dry regions. Good fatteners. Meat. Skins. About 75% of mated animals become pregnant. As a rule, only one kid is born. Birth weight is on average 2.4 kg.

Breed history: Indigenous breed of East Africa, which has been greatly improved in recent years for early maturity and fast growth. It is proof that, even in Third World countries, outstanding results can be achieved in animal breeding without external influence.

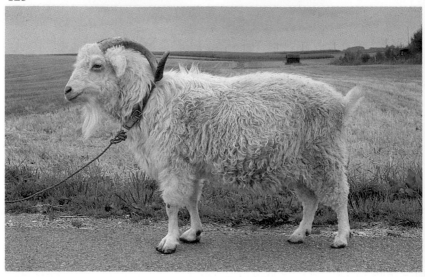

Angora

Characteristics: Pure white, with long, silky, curly hair. Slightly concave nose line. Medium-length to long lop ears. The males have corkscrew-shaped horns, curving back and out. The sickle-shaped horns of the females are considerably shorter.

	Male	Female
Height at shoulder	60	50
Weight	45–55	30–40

Distribution: Turkey (country of origin), South Africa, Lesotho, the USA, the former Soviet Union, Australia. Some animals in the former Federal Republic of Germany.
Uses: The Angora is mainly used for wool, which is sold as mohair. The world production of mohair wool is about 15,000 tonnes. Two fleeces per year. Annual wool yield 3–4 kg (females), 4–5 kg (males). Sensitive to

the cold; not really suitable for central Europe. Moderately prolific; only just over 80% of the females kid. Mature late. Single kids are usual; only 1% of births are twins. The females are considered poor mothers. The males are placid even in the mating season.
Breed history: This breed was originally kept in the province of Ankara (= Angora) on the Anatolian Plain. It is conceivable that there may have been Angora goats in the Near East for thousands of years; a passage in the fourth chapter of Solomon's Song of Songs in the Old Testament can be interpreted in this way. In the middle of the last century, Angora goats were taken to the USA, and later to other countries with suitable climates. Here, great improvements have since been made in the quality and quantity of the wool by selective breeding.

Horses

In central Europe, the horse can no longer be considered as agricultural livestock. It is used only for sport and leisure. This fact makes it easy to forget the important part played by the horse in the development of human civilisation and culture. Its strength and willingness to work made it invaluable in agriculture. It helped to work the land and reap the harvest, it took the agricultural products to town and facilitated more extensive trade between countries. Where commerce and transport were possible without horses, for instance where rivers allowed travel by ship, horses still had to be used to move the ships back up-river. For our eastern neighbours, the horse has not lost much of its original importance.

World-wide, it is not so numerous as cattle, sheep and pigs, but it occurs everywhere. It is kept in the tropics, occurs in its most improved form in deserts and survives north of the Arctic Circle, even when kept outdoors all year round. Horses thrive even if the grazing is so sparse that they must spend up to 14 hours a day looking for fodder, and drinking water is several days walk away. In unfavourable circumstances they will eat salty seaweed on the coast, and even fish that have been washed up.

Most horses are kept in countries where there is great reliance on agriculture, and where mechanisation is not universal or the use of horses is considered more economical. Other centres of horse-keeping are found in countries which, because of the standard of living, can afford to keep numerous horses as a pastime, or where large areas are suitable only for pasture (e.g. the USA). Horses can be used in many ways. Special uses require special breeding. This is the reason for the multiplicity of horse breeds.

Discussion on the evolution of the horse is still continuing. Experts who have studied this question extensively are, however, in no doubt that all domestic horses – from the tiny Falabella to the giant Shire – can be traced back to one ancient form (Herre and Röhrs, 1973; Hemmer, 1983). Views are not so unanimous on the question of which wild form is the ancestor of the domestic horse. Sometimes it is assumed that when the horse was domesticated there was only one single wild horse species, even if it had several different sub-species: the Przewalski horse (*Equus przewalskii*). There are about 200 examples of this horse species in captivity, and there may also be remnants in the area to which it has retreated – Mongolia, near the Chinese border. The upright mane of these horses is characteristic (**187**). They resemble all other wild horses in this feature. In contrast, no form of domestic horse has an upright mane, even if this is occasionally claimed to be the case. In the case of some breeds, for example the Fjord, the mane is often trimmed fashionably, but such an upright mane is then an artificial creation. Even in the case of the new Tarpan, a supposedly wild horse, the standing mane has not recurred, despite occasional cross-breeding with Przewalski horses.

The view that the original form of the domestic horse is to be found not in the Przewalski but in another species of wild horse is supported in particular by the different number of chromosomes: while the Przewalski has 66 chromosomes, domestic horses have only 64. All other differences – coloration, size, body proportions, etc. – can be regarded as resulting from domestication. The fact that the Tarpan was still regarded as a wild horse in the eighteenth century does not mean much. At that time, biological knowledge and understanding of the processes of domestication were not adequate for differentiating between truly wild animals and feral animals. Therefore the Tarpan may well have been a feral horse. It should be borne in mind that the Dülmen is still occasionally called a wild horse.

Man has always had a different relationship with horses from that with other agricultural livestock. This is probably not really due to the intelligence of these animals, on which opinions differ, in any case. However, it cannot be denied that they have a distinct sensibility and the ability to adjust to people and to react to the slightest utterance. The reason for the special relationship between man and horse is probably that the usefulness of the horse lies not in products but in its capabilities in conjunction with man. The ability to keep and own a horse was a distinction in the past. The expressions 'cavalier' and 'chivalrous' still bear witness to the high social prestige once enjoyed by the horse-rider.

Riding sports such as polo and arena riding are considered to be high points of court and village life all over the world. In the past, they were an essential part of the culture of a nation. Riding sports were not regarded merely as sport and pleasure. Aspects of character were practised and confirmed in them. In China, good polo players were given preference for ministerial posts in the past, as it was assumed that the skills learned in the game would be of value in performing their tasks (Isenbart and Bührer, 1969). The horses which achieved most success in competition were preferred for breeding. The result is not just the English thoroughbred and trotter but also numerous other breeds, such as the Quarter Horse and the Appaloosa. It is not at all rare for good sports horses to be descended from horses which have had a hard struggle for existence. In extensive cattle farming, some horses reveal a distinct 'cow sense'. This means they have the ability to comprehend their task in separating individual animals and to recognise their attempts to escape. Such horses can work quite independently without much assistance from the rider (124). It is difficult not to regard this ability as intelligence.

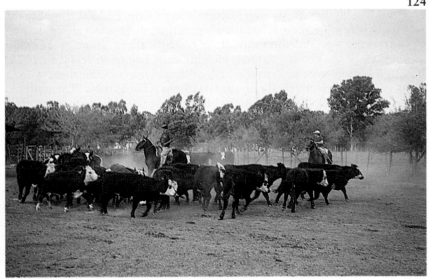

124 Cowherds sorting the animals in Argentina.

Table 12. Numbers of breeding horses in the Federal Republic of Germany in 1986.

Breed	Studs	Registered Mares	Total
Warmblood	1,348	52,321	53,669
Trakehner	243	3,221	3,464
Coldblood	151	2,084	2,235
English Thoroughbred	113	2,135	2,254
Trotter	383	3,728	4,111
Arab	618	3,728	4,346
Haflinger	348	6,682	7,030
German Riding Pony	281	4,261	4,542
Welsh Pony	264	1,793	2,057
Shetland Pony	257	1,352	1,609
Icelandic Pony	194	2,242	2,436
Fjordpferd	88	1,016	1,104
New Forest Pony	56	487	543
Connemara Pony	41	373	414
Dartmoor Pony	11	64	75
Other	160	626	786
Total	4,964	82,385	87,349

Source: 1986 annual report of the Deutsche Reiterliche Vereinigung e.V. (German Equestrian Association), and 1984 commercial report of the Association of Breeders and Friends of Warmbloods of Trakhener Stock e.V.

After World War II, the horse population in the Federal Republic of Germany was more than 1.5 million. After that, there was a sharp decline in horse keeping, and the population reached a low point of 252,000 animals in 1970. The subsequent increase ended again in 1981. In 1983, 354,000 horses were kept in the Federal Republic. In 1986 there were a total of 4964 selectively bred stud stallions (**Table 12**). Warmbloods (cross-breeds) and Arabs accounted for almost half of all stallions. The population of breeding mares was 87,349. While the main area for breeding warmbloods is around Hanover, in the case of ponies, most breeding mares are in Westphalia and Bavaria. In 1984 there were 17 auctions of riding horses in West Germany, at which 870 riding horses were sold at prices between 4,000 and 180,000 DM. The total turnover was DM 15.76 million and the average price of all riding horses sold was DM 18,120. There were 16,500 horses exported. Most of them went for slaughter (11,844), almost exclusively to France and Belgium. Breeding horses were bought mainly from the USA (367), and other types of working horse were bought primarily from Italy (2192) (source: FN annual report 1984). These examples show that the horse can have considerable commercial significance.

Unlike other species of livestock, there is no great difference between the sexes in horses. Stallions of individual breeds are only a few centimetres taller and only slightly heavier than the mares. Nevertheless, they can generally be recognised easily from the overall more compact build, the more powerful upper neck (stallion comb) and their temperament.

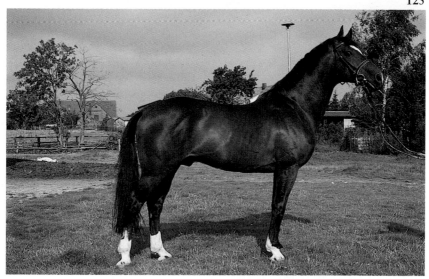

German Riding Horse

Characteristics: Generous lines. Epitome of warmblood horse. Expressive head. Powerful, well set-on neck. Prominent withers. Well-positioned shoulders. Deep chest. Compact body. Well muscled, sloping croup. Well set-on, nicely carried tail. Correct stance, strong leg bones. Hard hooves. All basic colours occur, with and without markings. Height 160–170 cm.

Distribution: The former West Germany. Occurs as a sporting and breeding horse in many other European countries as well as North and South America.

Uses: Good-natured, well-balanced. Strong nerves, good stamina. Its character and riding performance make it suitable for all types of riding. Outstanding multi-purpose horse, very willing. Leading breed all over the world for competition and dressage. Ideally suited as carriage and leisure horse.

Breed history: Warmbloods have been kept in Germany for many centuries. They resulted partly from crossing indigenous heavy horses with Andalusians, Neapolitans, oriental horses and thoroughbreds. The desire for a more elegant sporting horse in recent decades has meant that more thoroughbreds, Arabs and Trakehners have been used for cross-breeding. After World War II there was an increased exchange of blood between the individual associations, so the German warmblood breeds, which had originally differed in type, became increasingly homogeneous. In 1975 the horse breed societies decided to formulate a common breeding programme. The individual breed societies still have their own brand marks, however.

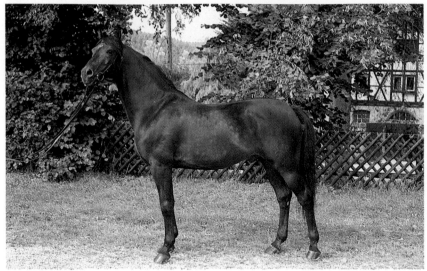

Trakehner

Characteristics: Very refined riding and sporting horse. Fine, expressive head. Long, curving neck. Long withers. Long, sloping shoulders. Long, deep, but rather narrow chest. Flat croup with high-set tail. Clean, sinewy limbs. Colours include black, brown, chestnut and grey. Stallions on average 165 cm, mares 162 cm high.

Distribution: Germany, Poland, former USSR, Netherlands and other European countries, North America and Africa.

Uses: Highly bred. Good stamina, fast. Long, lively gait. Limbs suitable for jumping and cross-country as well as dressage. Good temperament and excellent character. Matures late.

Breed history: In 1732 scattered stud farms were combined to form the Royal Trakehnen Stud Office, which later became the Central Trakehnen Stud. When the East Prussian Regional Studs were founded in 1787, Trakehnen was given the task of providing stud stallions for the Regional Horse Breeding Organisation. Prime stud animals now included only their own stallions, Arabs and thoroughbreds. The Arabs gave the Trakehners their beauty, the thoroughbreds gave them their large build, and both contributed to their good nerves and nobility. After World War I, they changed from cavalry horses to agricultural horses: fairly strong, good deep ribs and excellent temperament. At the end of World War II they moved to West Germany in a week-long trek which was full of privation. Thoroughbred stallions are used extensively. Other countries continue to breed mainly from the lines of Dampfross, Parcifal and Tempelhüter, etc. The Trakehner has made a considerable contribution to the refinement of other warmblood breeds. In Germany and elsewhere there are about 4,000 registered mares and about 300 registered stallions.

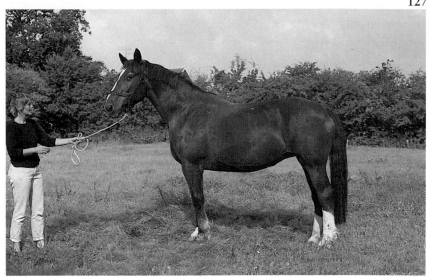

East Friesian

Characteristics: Heaviest German warmblood breed. Mainly black or brown with few markings. Head not too large. Neck quite long and set high. Long, sloping, well-muscled shoulders. Medium-length, flexible back. Saddle position well marked. Croup long, slightly sloping and well-muscled. Deep body. Well-knit flanks. Strong constitution with powerful but clean joints. Height 160–165 cm.

Distribution: The old East Friesian breed range. In the past also found in Hesse, Saxony and Silesia.

Uses: Calm temperament. Because of its size it is suitable as a draught horse on the heavy land of East Friesland. Impressive show horse. Frugal, matures early. Lively movement with a long stride.

Breed history: It was developed from land strains by crossing with oriental, English and Normandy stock. Later it was strongly influenced by the heavy Hanoverian and, owing to cooperation with the Oldenburg breed area, the Oldenburg. During the period when it was changing from a draught horse to a riding horse after World War II, Arab thoroughbreds were used extensively to give the East Friesian nobility and toughness. The East Friesian stud book later became linked to the society of Hanoverian warmblood breeders. Today, East Friesian riding horses are bred on pure Hanoverian stock. There are few remaining examples of the original East Friesian. Attempts are now being made to preserve the remaining breeding stock as a 'heavy warmblood' by using Oldenburgs and an English Cleveland Bay stallion.

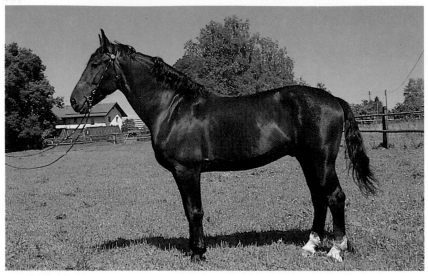

Oldenburg

Characteristics: Well-balanced heavy warmblood. Brown, dark brown or black with few markings. Harmonious and muscular build. Good neck conformation. Head generally compressed. Strong constitution. Height 157–165 cm, weight 550–650 kg.

Distribution: Only a few remaining examples in the old Oldenburg core breeding area. Somewhat more widely distributed in the subsequent traditional breeding areas such as Poland and the former German Democratic Republic (Moritzburg).

Uses: Flexible, willing. Elegant, heavy carriage horse with typical reliable draught and working qualities. Calm temperament. Energetic, effective trotting gait. Tough, robust and resistant to harsh weather.

Breed history: It was developed by mating Friesian mares with Andalusian and oriental stallions. The 'elegant Oldenburg carriage horse' was one of the oldest and most highly bred warmblood breeds in Germany. In the seventeenth century, the historian V. Halem wrote: 'the Oldenburg horses are bought for their size, beauty and strength and are prized by Counts and potentates'. From the middle of the 1930s, English thoroughbreds and Anglo-Normans were crossed with them. The breeding plan protected the Oldenburg breed type for a long time, but during its conversion to a riding horse in the 1960s and 1970s by means of extensive use of thoroughbred and Hanoverian stallions, the original type had to be displaced. Breeding of warmbloods in the Netherlands and Denmark can be traced back essentially to Oldenburg stock. The same applies to the breeding of heavy warmbloods in Austria. About 100 years ago, Oldenburg stallions were introduced into the old breeding area of the Rottal, so the last remaining Rottals resemble the Oldenburg.

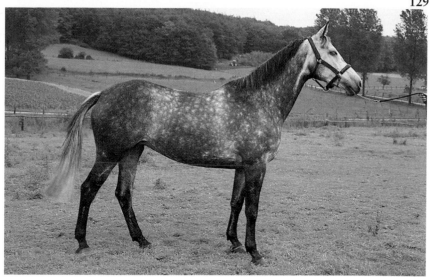

Senne

Characteristics: Light, elegant, medium-sized warmblood of Anglo-Arab type. Currently mainly brown and grey. Height 155–165 cm.

Distribution: Native to the 'Senne', an extensive heath area on the southern slope of the Teutoburg Forest between Bielefeld and Paderborn.

Uses: Used mainly as a riding horse, but also suitable as a carriage horse. Hardy, contented and frugal. Pleasant temperament. Matures late.

Breed history: One of the oldest German horse breeds; first mentioned in 1160. Until 1680 the stud was near Detmold; then it was moved to Lopshorn. The true habitat of the Senne was forest and heath; it lived outdoors all year round. Mares and foals were only rounded up to select the necessary animals for work and riding. From the middle of the eighteenth century, stallions of foreign descent, mainly refined horses of Spanish or oriental origin, were crossed with them. From 1870 the horses were no longer driven to forest pasture; they thus lost the basis for their physical and temperamental specialisation.

After World War I the remaining horses passed from the ownership of the Princes of Lippe to that of the Association of Lippe Horse Breeders. In 1935 the stud was disbanded. A Dutch woman, Mrs J. M. Immink, obtained some of the animals and continued breeding them on Lopshorn. In 1946 the stud was finally disbanded. The horses were sold to private individuals and institutions in the former West Germany and the Netherlands. Here some have continued to be bred in accordance with the original breeding plan.

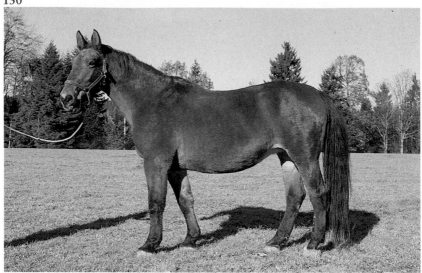

Rottal

Characteristics: Medium-sized, powerful, low-slung carriage and cart horse. Predominantly brown with few markings; less frequently black. Powerful neck. Well-developed facial area. Large, intelligent eyes. Well set-on, medium-length neck. Reasonably long withers. Deep and broad chest; well-sprung ribs. Round, longish, slightly sloping croup. Nicely carried tail, set fairly high. Clean, powerful joints. Well-formed hooves. Height 160–165 cm.

Distribution: Rottal and surrounding areas. Occasionally in the rest of Bavaria.

Uses: Versatile commercial horse. Eminently suitable for the needs of agriculture in the past, but also ideal for all types of equestrian sports. It was called the 'Rottal carriage horse' in the past, which indicates its main application. Good temperament. Long, lively, energetic gait. Good stamina and flexibility. Reasonably prolific and long-lived.

Breed history: The Rottal horse breed is the earliest mentioned historically in Germany, apart from the East Friesian. In Rottal in Lower Bavaria it was bred on the basis of Hungarian Raid horses with Arabian stock from the tenth century. In the eighteenth century, Holstein and Anglo-Norman stallions were used to introduce size and strength into the breed. At the end of the nineteenth century, more refined Oldenburg stallions played a decisive part in the development of the breed. In recent decades, Hanoverians, Trakehners, thoroughbreds and Arabs have been used to transform the type into a versatile high-performance horse. Currently there are only about 30 mares with at least 50% Rottal blood.

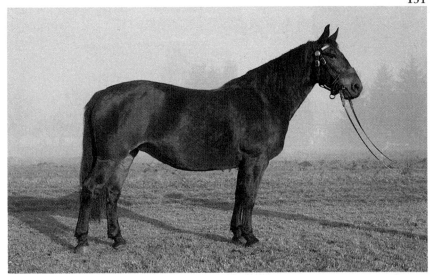

Old Württemberg

Characteristics: Medium-sized, compact horse of the cob type, but quite elegant. Good breadth and depth to body. Relatively short legs. Clean constitution with well-formed joints. Strong bones. Hard hooves. Height 160–165 cm.

Distribution: Originally distributed over the whole of Württemberg, with Oberland and Schwäbische Alb the breeding centres. Only a few animals are left.

Uses: Frugal. Hard and robust. Willing. Strong nerves, obliging. Excellent draught animal. Good stamina. Versatile. Suitable for agriculture and as a carriage horse for medium-sized loads. Long, lively gait.

Breed history: Although the main city of Württemberg (Stuttgart = stud garden) must always have had a close relationship with the horse, and has a horse on its coat of arms, Württemberg has never produced a native breed of its own. The characteristics of the Württemberg warmblood in the last century were produced mainly by the Anglo-Norman, especially by the stallion 'Faust' which was bought as a three-year-old in Normandy for 5800 Marks. Mares also came from Holstein, Hungary, Carinthia and other regions. In 1908 the first stud book was opened, and 406 mares were entered in it initially. From the 1930s, of all the stallions used only Arabs and to a limited extent, Trakehners, proved suitable. After World War I the breed was established in form and characteristics. Later, a great effort to improve the breed involved displacement crossbreeding with East Prussians. Now there are only a few animals which have not been transformed into elegant riding horses and which still embody the heavier Old Württemberg in the type of the Anglo-Norman.

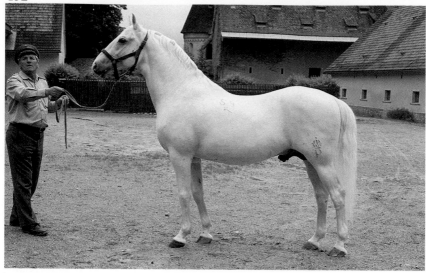

Lipizzaner

Characteristics: The body shape corresponds to that of the grand baroque horse. Most Lipizzaners are white. Occasionally there are brown, black and chestnut animals; they are not used for breeding, however. The foals are born black, grey or brown. Pleasant, expressive, often convex head. Intelligent eyes. The neck is powerful, set high and nobly carried. Powerful, muscular back. Strong croup. The well set-on tail is thick and composed of fine hair. The distinctly short limbs are clean and shapely; they have clean hocks and well-formed hooves. Height 155–167 cm, weight 450–550 kg.

Distribution: Austria, Hungary, Yugoslavia. Smaller numbers in many other European countries.

Uses: Distinguished by hardiness, stamina and contentedness. Frugal. Quick to learn, intelligent and docile. Natural high knee action. Particularly suitable as a riding and training horse as well as a carriage horse. Matures very late, long-lived. Lipizzaners are the horses used in the Spanish Riding School in Vienna.

Breed history: Spanish horses came from the Iberian peninsula to Lipica (now in Yugoslavia) in 1580. They were bought repeatedly in the eighteenth century and, since about 1700, Italian, German and Danish horses have been introduced to improve them. In the middle of the nineteenth century they were crossed with Arabs. After a temporary stay in Kladruby in Czechoslovakia, the horses were taken to the Federal Stud in Piber in Styria in 1920, where they have remained since. Occasionally Arabs are crossed with them.

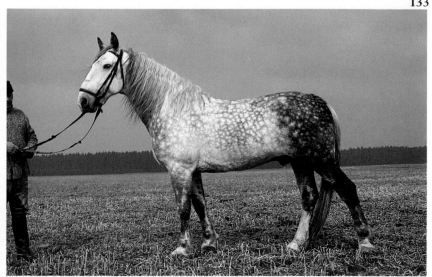

Kladruber

Characteristics: Baroque strain of draught horse; somewhat heavier than the Lipizzaner. Grey or black. Distinctly convex head. Large, round eyes. Arched, short neck. Wide chest. Long, soft back. Relatively short, broad croup. Muscular legs. Flexible fetlocks. Height 160–170 cm.

Distribution: Czechoslovakia, Austria. Some animals in the former Federal Republic of Germany.

Uses: Good-natured and willing. Powerful cart horse with high, short strides. Good show horse. Successful in dressage. In Czechoslovakia it is used to improve land races. Matures late.

Breed history: Its ancestors came from Spain in the sixteenth century. The Court Stud at Kladruby, founded in 1562, bred this heavy warmblood as a coach horse, intended for the Royal Stables of the Austrian Emperor. Occasionally, Hungarian and Italian (Neapolitan) stallions were used to refresh the stock. The latter included the founder of the grey line. After 1800, little outside stock was used for cross-breeding. Before World War I they were more than 180 cm high, but later they were bred for a more manageable size. Since the decline of the original use, the breed base has become very narrow. It includes little more than 100 brood mares and ten stud stallions. The different colours are bred separately: the greys in Kladrub, the blacks in Slatinany. To prevent inbreeding resulting from the small numbers of this breed, Lipizzaners and recently also a Friesian stallion are used occasionally. Kladruber stallions were two of the founders of the Lipizzaner line.

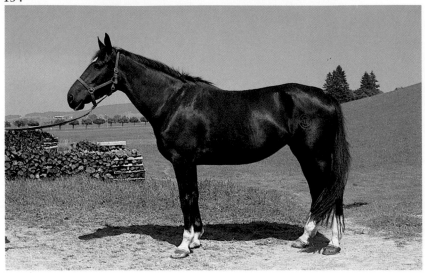

Einsiedler

Characteristics: Powerfully built, light warmblood. Well proportioned with expressive face. Strong shoulders. Deep chest. Powerful hindquarters. Height 156–165 cm. All basic colours occur; bays are the most common, chestnuts are less frequent. Blacks and greys are rare.

Distribution: The main population is at the Einsiedeln monastery in the canton of Schwyz. There are isolated animals throughout Switzerland.

Uses: Versatile, all-round horse. Excellent for the saddle and for harness. Light, elegant movements. Sometimes good jumpers. Obedient and of impeccable character.

Breed history: The breed got its name from the Benedictine Abbey of Einsiedeln. The first reference to it dates from 1064. This breed had its golden age in the sixteenth century. Around 1800 the number of horses at the monastery fell owing to the effects of war. It was therefore necessary to purchase animals from the surrounding area to preserve the stock. As the breed nevertheless reached a low point about the middle of the nineteenth century, foreign stallions were used in the second half of the century: initially a Yorkshire stallion, later Anglo-Normans, which had a formative influence on the type of the breed. Einsiedlers were used at first for travel and transport. Later they were also very popular in the Swiss cavalry. They were particularly prized in Upper Italy. About 20 years ago it was decided to develop the breed into a modern riding horse. This was achieved mainly with French stallions. In Einsiedeln itself there are now about 20 brood mares. The Einsiedlers have their own brand: a raven in flight with the letter E in a circle.

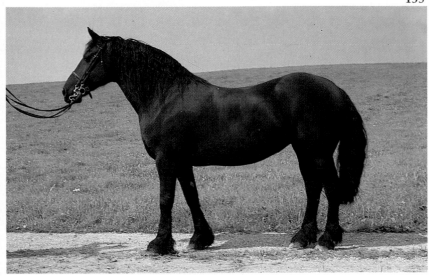

Friesian

Characteristics: Heavy warmblood. Always black. Relatively small head with small ears. The prominent neck is carried high. It is slightly curved (swan-neck) and has a long mane. The back is fairly short, the withers are not overdeveloped. It has a powerful constitution. There is prominent feather on the pasterns. On average it is 155–160 cm high.

Distribution: Netherlands, mainly the province of Friesland. Large population in South Africa. The main population in the former West Germany is in North–Rhine/Westphalia.

Uses: Energetic, high trotting action. Smooth gait. In the past it was used mainly in agriculture, today it is primarily used as a carriage horse. Contented and docile.

Breed history: Old Dutch breed, which was cross-bred with Spanish horses in the sixteenth and seventeenth centuries. In accordance with the taste of the age, it was bred as a 'baroque' horse. Friesians already had a good reputation as strong but elegant riding horses, which were suitable for classical dressage. About 100 years later, when trotting races were popular in the Netherlands, they proved to be fast sprinters over short distances (300–600 m). When, in the nineteenth century, they could no longer compete with the German breeds of the same line of development which were then better, their breeding plan was changed completely – essentially by introducing English blood.

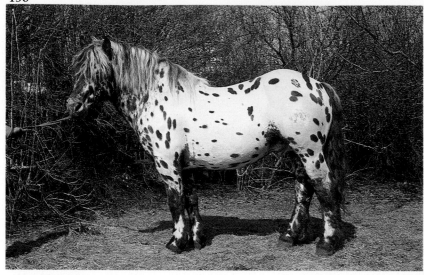

Knapstruper

Characteristics: Heavy warmblood. Exclusively white with black spots. The long hair and the lower parts of the legs can be white or dark. Convex head. Broad neck. Deep chest. Well-muscled. Powerful constitution. Height 160 cm.
Distribution: Denmark. Isolated animals in other European countries.
Uses: Predominantly used as circus and trick-riding horses.
Breed history: This breed is traced back to a refined mare of unknown origin which a Spanish officer sold in Denmark at the beginning of the nineteenth century. Contrary to the original intention, the mare was not slaughtered but came into the ownership of a breeder of Frederiksborg horses and thus to the Knapstrup estate. This mare was a spiky-haired sable chestnut whose long hair was white and which had numerous white spots on the loins. Her offspring included a large number of piebald horses, which were formed into a breed. Since the middle of the nineteenth century, other breeds have continually been crossed with it, mainly the Frederiksborg, with which it finally largely merged. In addition to the characteristic coloration, it still differs from the latter by being somewhat lighter. It is kept primarily on the island of Seeland.

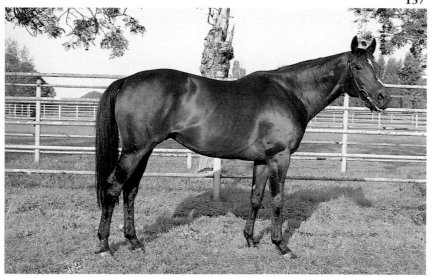

English Thoroughbred

Characteristics: With this breed, it is not the appearance of a horse which decides its use in breeding, but its performance. Square conformation. Most animals are brown or dark brown, but other colours occur. Clean, fine head with large, clear eyes. Long, muscular neck. Sloping shoulders. Prominent, high withers. Back of medium length. Powerful, long and muscular croup. Powerful constitution with short cannons and firm, hard hooves. Silky coat. Long hair is very fine. The average height is 160–170 cm, and the weight is 400–500 kg.

Distribution: Distributed world-wide. Outside the UK, it has been most significant in the USA, France, Italy and the former Federal Republic of Germany.

Uses: Extremely fast, especially in middle distances, both on the flat and in steeplechases. When their career on the track is over, they are often used for equestrian sports and dressage. They are particularly useful for improving many other breeds.

Breed history: All English Thoroughbreds can be traced back essentially to three oriental stallions (Byerley Turk, Darley Arabian and Godolphin Barb) and nearly 50 mares. The publication of the 'General Stud Book' in England in 1793 had a decisive influence on the consolidation of this breed. Horses to be entered into it must have, in addition to suitable ancestry among close relatives, proof of acceptable performance on the race track, which affirms confidence that they are pure bred. The English Thoroughbred has been involved in the formation of most warm-blood breeds. It is also still crossed with them repeatedly to maintain their nobility, toughness and nerve. International abbreviation: xx.

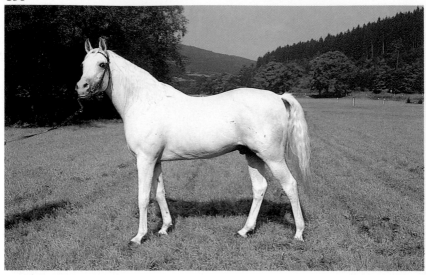

Arab Thoroughbred

Characteristics: The most refined breed of horse. All colours occur. The most common is white in all possible shades. Black animals are rare. The small, fine head is carried high and free. The forehead is noticeably broad and high. The head narrows considerably towards the muzzle. The bridge of the nose is slightly dished at the transition to the facial part of the head. Large, flared nostrils. Small, alert ears. Large, expressive, protruding eyes. Short back line. Elegantly carried tail. Nicely shaped joints and clearly defined tendons. Very hard hooves. The skin and long hair are fine and silky. No feather on the legs. Height 145–155 cm. Fully grown animals weigh 400–450 kg.

Distribution: Distributed almost all over the world. Originally found in the countries of the Arabian peninsula as well as Egypt. Significant populations in the USA; in Europe, particularly common in the UK, the Netherlands and the former Eastern Bloc countries.

Uses: Famed for its stamina, contented nature and fast recovery after great exertion. It has courage, high intelligence and a placid temperament. It takes the saddle well, but is also capable of carrying heavy loads for long distances. Matures late. Long-lived.

Breed history: Among Arab horses, only those which have always been bred within lines which go back to a specific ancient stock are Arab Thoroughbreds; pure breeding and often in-breeding were always carried out. The first occurrence of this horse is not known. It is certain that in the seventh century Mohammed was not the founder, but merely the great patron of this breed. Introduced to the non-Arab world in the nineteenth century. In its countries of origin it has declined sharply since mechanisation.

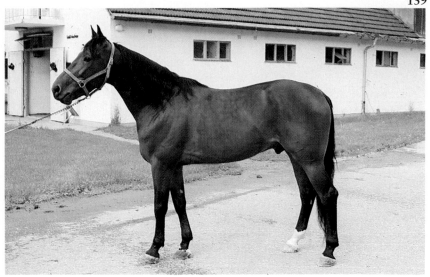

Trotter

Characteristics: In general, longer but somewhat smaller and with a finer constitution than the English Thoroughbred. It does however have a strong bone structure. There are brown, chestnut, and black animals, and also lighter colours. The rear quarters are well developed and somewhat higher than the withers (trotter's croup). It weighs between 450 and 600 kg, height 152–163 cm.

Distribution: World-wide.

Uses: Trotters compete in races in which they generally have to cover a distance of between 1600 and 2400 m at a trot. Trotting is defined as a gait with a diagonal hoot sequence, in which the front foot and rear foot of opposite sides are lifted from the ground simultaneously and replaced simultaneously. The world record is 1:11.3 min for 1 km. The German record of 1:15.5 min is held by the stallion Simmerl. Trotters are sometimes also used as carriage horses.

Breed history: The German Trotter breed has an American base; it was also influenced by the French Trotter after World War II. The American Trotter's ancestry includes the English Thoroughbred, Arabs and pacers of various breeds. The French Trotter is descended essentially from the Anglo-Norman. Only in its country of origin does it have greater significance.

The sport of trotting developed only after 1874 in Germany; the Trotter was bred there from 1885. Before World War II, Germany was a leader in trotting. Although German Trotter breeding has produced first-class stallions in recent decades which have sired excellent offspring (e.g. Permit), it still depends on the introduction of foreign blood.

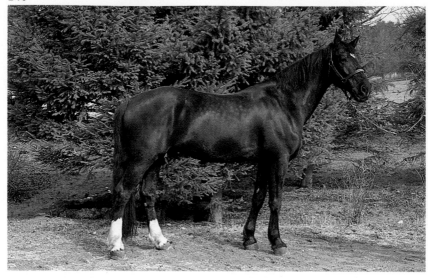

Orlov Trotter

Characteristics: Powerful, compact horse. Considerably heavier than American and French Trotters. Large head. Large eyes. Short ears. Well set-on, arched neck. Powerful back. Broad, slightly sloping croup. Strong leg bones. Often pronounced feather on the pasterns. All basic colours occur. Height 160–165 cm.

Distribution: Former Soviet Union. Other former Eastern Bloc countries. Small numbers in central Europe.

Uses: Has good stamina. Long-lived. Prolific. Excellent carriage and sleigh horse. In racing it is distinctly inferior to the other trotting breeds. Well suited to equestrian sports.

Breed history: Count Alexei Grigory-evich Orlov took part in a coup in which Catherine II came to the Russian throne. She later gave him a large estate among the enormous steppe lands of the province of Voronesh. Count Orlov, a great lover of horses, obtained many Turkish, Persian and Arabian horses from far-flung areas of the Russian Empire. The splendid Arab Smetanka, which he bought for 60,000 gold roubles — a fortune in those days — was brought to his Ostrov estate near Moscow. Bars I, a grandson of the stallion Smetanka, in whose veins also flowed Dutch and Danish blood of Spanish/Andalusian descent, was an exceedingly good trotter. He was the progenitor of the Orlov Trotters which have Danish, Dutch, Norfolk Trotter and English Thoroughbred blood. The desire was for a fast, elegant coach horse. The first regular trotting races in western Europe involved Orlov Trotters exclusively. As a working horse for pulling coaches or sleighs it had to be sufficiently well-built and strong to withstand the great demands made on it.

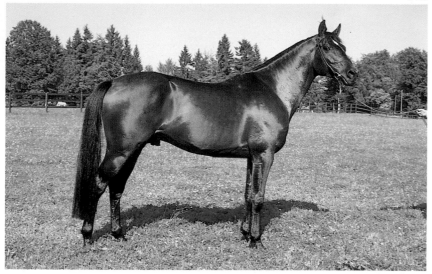

Anglo-Arab

Characteristics: Pleasant appearance. Refined. In the past, a light horse, often of fine conformation. Today a better calibre is required. All basic colours occur; brown predominates. Nice head. Neck well set-on. Prominent withers. Long, sloping shoulders. Good depth and breadth. Clean, well-defined legs. Height 160–170 cm.

Distribution: High–performance horse with excellent basic gaits and outstanding jumping ability. It is used with success in all equestrian events from dressage and show jumping to all-round tests and steeplechasing, and has won many important international prizes.

Breed history: The Anglo-Arab was developed by crossing Arab and English Thoroughbreds, as the name indicates, and was intended to possess the advantages of both breeds. Consolidated studs. Originally developed independently in France, Poland and Spain. In the former Federal Republic of Germany, the Anglo-Arab Ramses (v. Rittersporn), for example, has earned a good reputation. His offspring include many famous show jumpers and dressage horses.

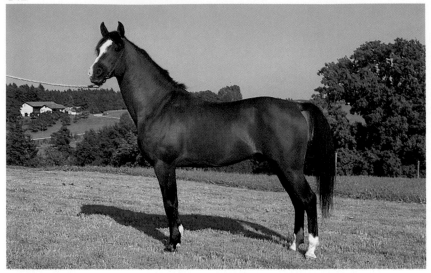

Shagya

Characteristics: An Arab with a larger build and with more riding horse features. All colours occur. Greys predominate; blacks are rare. There may be white markings on the head and the lower extremities. Fine Arab head. Well-developed jaws. Large nostrils. Well-muscled, nicely set-on neck. Tail carried high ('pheasant–like'). Stallions 156–165 cm high, mares 153–160 cm.

Distribution: Hungary, Czechoslovakia, the former Soviet Union, Austria, the former Federal Republic of Germany, Denmark, Switzerland, the USA.

Uses: Excellent, versatile saddle and carriage horse. Eminently rideable. Outstanding movements. Enormous jumping ability. Tough and has stamina. Suitable for long-distance riding or for hunting with the pack.

Breed history: Developed in the nineteenth century in the Hungarian military studs of the Imperial and Royal Monarchy from desert Arabs by cross-breeding with indigenous land races, Andalusians, Lipizzaners and English Thoroughbreds. The desire was for a horse of the size and calibre of a cavalry or carriage horse, but which would also be an excellent show horse. The Royal Guard in Budapest rode fine Shagya Arabs. This breed was further developed by pure breeding, with the best and finest-looking desert Arabs being used from time to time, so that the breed would not get too heavy. Recognised by the World Arab Organisation as 'Pure-Bred Shagya Arab' since 1978. Systematic breeding has been conducted in central Europe since 1960; in the former Federal Republic of Germany, the regional centre is in the north. There are only a few hundred registered brood animals. Named after 'Shagya', the founder of the line, a thoroughbred Arab imported into Hungary in 1837.

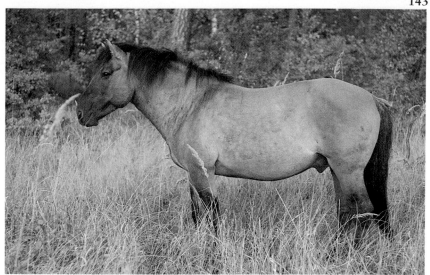

Polish Konik

Characteristics: Powerful, well-muscled pony. Slightly top-heavy. Firm back. Short, sloping croup. Relatively undeveloped chest. The colour is brown, dark bay or mousy grey, often with a black line along the back. There are often zebra stripes on the legs. The mane, forelock and tail are well developed. Height 120–140 cm, weight 280–370 kg.

Distribution: Poland. Some animals in the former West Germany (East Friesland).

Uses: Robust. Able to withstand cold weather. Very contented. Good draught animal. Strong bones, very hard hooves.

Breed history: Konik means 'little horse' in Polish. In Germany this breed was also known by the name Panje horse. It derives from a primitive land race, the Mierzyn (i.e. Middle horse). Planned breeding started about 1927 in Poland. After World War II, several studs were set up to develop the breed, and Koniks are also kept in several research institutes. Fjord horses were cautiously crossed with them for a while. In 1936, on the initiative of T. Vetulani, some selected Koniks of the wild horse type were allowed to range freely in the hope of recreating the ancient type by means of appropriate selection. Today there are such horses in various reserves and stations. They are very uniform in type and coloration; steely grey predominates, with almost no brown (the designation mousy grey is misleading). In the game stud at Popielno in the Mazury, several herds are allowed to range freely all year round on a reserve of 320 hectares. Contrary to expectations, they have not become wild, but positively friendly. Some of these horses are used in agriculture.

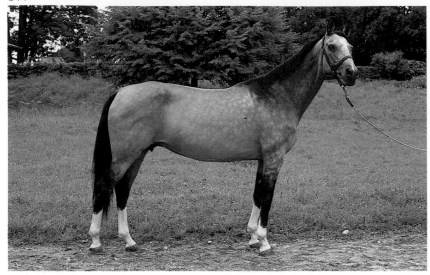

Akhal-Tekke

Characteristics: Very refined horse. The most common colours are golden bay, dun, isabelline and black; there are also greys and chestnuts. The legs are long and the girth shallow. Straight, strong back with long, high withers. Long body. Fine, clean limbs with well-defined tendons. Small, hard hooves. The skin and hair are extremely fine and have a characteristic golden sheen. The long hair is fine. Three types are classified in the stud book: standard, middle and heavy. Height 152–164 cm.

Distribution: The main breeding centres are in the steppe regions of the southern former Soviet Union and in northern Iran. Also found in the former West Germany and other central European countries.

Uses: Real desert horses. Refined. Tough. Good stamina. Tolerant of heat. Elegant, light movements. Energetic and temperamental with a good stride and a long, supple gait in a gallop. Well suited to dressage, but also excellent show jumpers. In addition they are good all-round and long-distance horses. Impressive endurance.

Breed history: Named after the oasis of Akhal and the Turkmenian people of the Tekke, who live on the northern slopes of the Kopet–Dag mountains. Planned breeding has been carried out for several centuries. It has been registered in the state stud book since 1934–35. The Akhal–Tekke had a great influence on the development of warmblood breeds in many parts of the world; in Germany, it influenced the Trakehner considerably. There are about 1500 animals in all. Breeding is based on about 300 mares. The current breeding centre is the Makhmud–Kuli stud in the Akhal oasis near Ashkhabad. There are about 120 animals of this breed in the former Federal Republic of Germany.

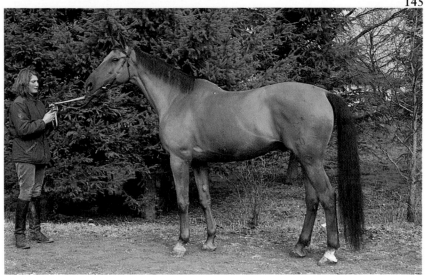

Don

Characteristics: Stately, light, but powerful horse of the thoroughbred type. Low build. Predominantly chestnut with a distinct golden sheen. Medium-sized, fine head. Well-spaced eyes. Fairly small ears. Long, straight neck. Good withers. Broad back. Powerful hindquarters. Clean constitution. Height 160–165 cm.

Distribution: The former Soviet Union. Other East European countries. There are also a few examples in the former Federal Republic of Germany.

Uses: Tough and with unusual stamina. Undemanding. Tolerant of harsh weather. Outstanding coach horse and first-class riding horse. In 1883, four officers and 14 Cossacks rode 1300 km from Novgorod to Moscow in 11 days in temperatures as low as −20°C. In 1950, five Don horses covered 305 km within 24 hours; another, Zenit, covered 311.6 km.

Breed history: Derived from the horses of the Tartars. Originally the favourite horse of the Don Cossacks in pony size. In 1770, the Cossack Ataman M. I. Platov founded the first stud on the Don. In the nineteenth century it achieved a larger build by crossbreeding with English Thoroughbreds, Orlov Trotters and other Russian breeds. It lives in the steppes of the southern former USSR under very harsh conditions — outdoors all year round on sparse fodder. In World War II, the valuable brood horses of this breed were evacuated beyond the Urals. Subsequently, the breed has been rebuilt systematically, developing from a cavalry horse into a versatile warmblood horse. Breeding centres are in the Don region, Kirghiz and in Kazakhstan. Don horses from Issyk–Kul have the best reputation; this is the most easterly stud in the former Soviet Union, situated at an altitude of 1600 m in the Tien Shan mountains.

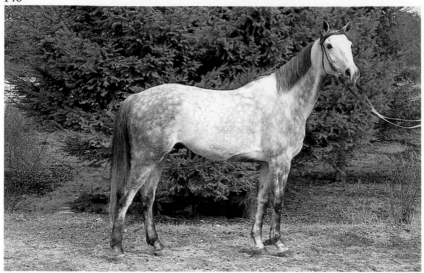

Tersk

Characteristics: Elegant riding horse of the Arab type, but with a larger frame. Light grey or white horses with a silver sheen, more rarely chestnut or bay. Elegant, Arab head with a straight or slightly concave nose line. Broad forehead. Large, expressive eyes. Long, pointed ears. Long, elegantly carried neck. Prominent withers. Long back with powerful renal area. Tail high set-on. Clean legs with strong bones. Skin has a distinct silvery sheen. Height 154–162 cm, occasionally higher.

Distribution: The former Soviet Union. Increasing numbers in central Europe.

Uses: Good cross-country horse. Has stamina. Used for flat racing with good results. Excellent all-round horse. Impressive appearance, good dressage performance and gentle temperament have led to its use in the circus. Elegant, lively movements. Learns easily.

Breed history: In 1921, the Soviet state founded the state stud of Tersk on the Caucasian estates of Count Stroganoff and Sultan Girea. The basis of the breed was formed by the remnants of the well-known Streletzker, as well as Kabardins, cross-breeds, English Thoroughbreds, and Dons. The progenitors were the two pure-bred Arab stallions Cenitel and Cilindr. The breeding plan was initially to produce good riding horses for the army. From 1925 the desire was for an elegant, tough riding horse of the Arab type, but with a larger frame. As the breeding base had become narrow in the chaos of war, it was crossed with Dons, Kabardins and English Thoroughbreds after World War II. The aim of selective breeding was a type corresponding largely to the Arab, but somewhat larger and more muscular. The breed was officially recognised in 1948–49. Soon afterwards, the herd was moved to the state stud at Stavropol.

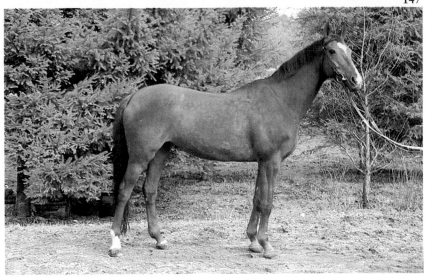

Budyonny

Characteristics: Robust, somewhat heavily built, but nevertheless an elegant riding horse. Predominantly chestnut, but other colours occur, except grey. Fine, clean head. Straight nose line. Small ears. Long, high-set, muscular neck. Strong shoulders. Prominent withers. Deep chest. Well-knit, strong loins. Powerful constitution. Fine coat with a golden sheen. Height generally 162–165 cm.

Distribution: The former Soviet Union. Smaller numbers in central Europe.

Uses: Undemanding. Good temperament and stamina. Well suited to all equestrian sports, especially long-distance and steeplechasing. The stallion Santos covered 1800 km in 15 days. The breed has also achieved good results in flat racing; the record for 2-year-olds over 1000 m is 1.03 min. Internationally it has achieved great success in show-jumping, dressage and military events.

Breed history: Named after Marshal Semyon Mikhailovich Budyonny, who signed the order to found new studs on the Salic steppes in 1921. The original aim was a first-class riding horse. Elite Don mares (the breeding centre was at Rostov on the Don plain) and Black Sea mares (horses of the Zaporog Cossacks) were mated with English Thoroughbred stallions. Strict selective breeding was performed from the outset. In 1941 the studs were evacuated beyond the Urals, from where they returned at the end of 1944 to 1945. The breed was consolidated after World War II. It was officially recognised in 1948. The horses are kept intentionally in large herds on pasture almost all year round. The powerful constitution and good condition are considered to result from the hardiness this engenders and to the healthy diet. Only when there is hard frost or deep snow are the herds protected from the wind.

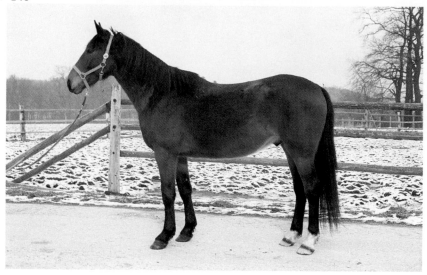

Kabardin

Characteristics: Powerful horse of medium build. Mostly brown, dark bay or black, rarely chestnut. The head has a straight nose line. Prominent withers. Powerful body. Fairly long back. Sloping croup (mountain horse). Clean constitution. Relatively short legs. Very hard hooves. Height 147–155 cm. Today there are also many Anglo-Kabardins which are somewhat larger.

Distribution: The former Soviet Union (Caucasus). The former Federal Republic of Germany.

Uses: Sure-footed. Good stamina. Tough. Willing. Undemanding. Long-lived and prolific. It is considered to be the best mountain breed in the former USSR. Placid temperament. Patient. Versatile. Suitable as a pack animal and for long-distance riding; 15 riders on Kabardins and Anglo–Kabardins covered 3000 km in the Caucasus in 47 days. Anglo–Kabardins are faster and better for dressage. Intelligent and with a good sense of orientation (even in darkness). The mares' milk is made into various products.

Breed history: The region of origin is Kabardin in the former Soviet Union. It presumably derives from the Circassian horse. Little is known of its origins otherwise. During the course of time it has been improved with Turkmenians, Karabakhs and Arabs. In the former Soviet Union it has also been widely distributed outside the Caucasus since the sixteenth century, and it still is. The main studs are Malokarakhayev and Malinskoye in the northern Caucasus.

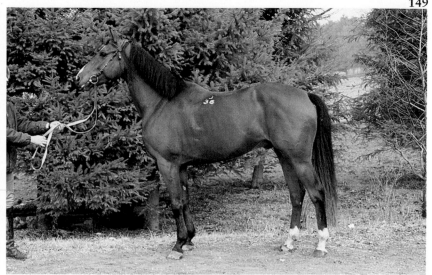

Karabai

Characteristics: It resembles the Arab in size and type, but is more powerful. Clean head. Broad back. Generally very muscular. Clean legs. The long hair is not very prominent. All basic colours occur. Height 148–152 cm, occasionally higher.

Distribution: The former Soviet Union (Uzbekistan). The former Federal Republic of Germany.

Uses: Good stamina, fast and agile. Undemanding. Intelligent and courageous. Very capable, willing to work and adaptable. In its native region it is used for the wildest equestrian games. Suitable for agricultural work. Used as a draught and pack horse in the mountains. Versatile.

Breed history: Ancient breed, which has probably been repeatedly crossed with horses belonging to the neighbouring peoples (Mongols, Kirghizians and Turkmenians). It was mentioned 2400 years ago. It was well-known and widely distributed in the eighteenth century. There are three types with differing constitutions, which are used for different purposes. The breeding centre is the Dshisak stud.

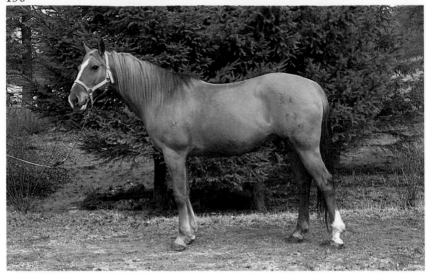

Karabakh

Characteristics: The build is at the lower end of the mid-range. Similar to the Arab. Refined head. Broad forehead. Prominent, large eyes. Narrow nose region. Small muzzle. Powerful, well-formed neck. Prominent withers. Compact, short body. Somewhat sloping croup. Clean, very fine constitution. Predominantly chestnut, but also dun, with a soft, silky coat with a golden sheen; rarely isabelline or grey. Height on average 150 cm.

Distribution: The former Soviet Union (Karabakh mountains, Azerbaijan), Iran. Isolated animals in the former Federal Republic of Germany.

Uses: Energetic. Tough. Light, nimble movements. Good riding horse. In its native country is considered to be an excellent horse for equestrian games.

Breed history: Ancient horse breed. Reference was made to it 1500 years ago. Presumably derives from refined Turkmenian, Persian and Arabian horses. Leading Russian horse experts consider the Karabakh to be the only breed which has been kept pure. In some ancient texts it is called the most refined horse breed. It had its golden age in the eighteenth century, when it was coveted all over Europe. It has been crossed with numerous other Russian breeds, especially the Don. When the Persians conquered Baku in 1826, they took almost all of the Karabakh herds as plunder. Queen Elizabeth II of England received the golden dun 'Zaman' from Nikita Khrushchev, and it produced outstanding offspring when used for breeding riding ponies in England. The Karabakh is now bred mainly in the Akdam stud in Azerbaijan. Occasionally it is still crossed with Arabs.

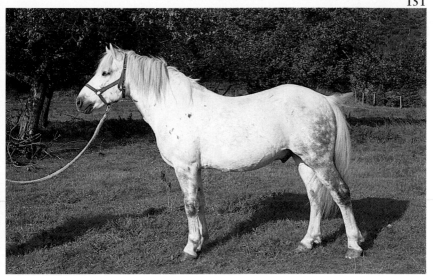

Camargue

Characteristics: The type is very reminiscent of the Berber. Adult animals are always grey. Short head with a straight nose profile, broad forehead and small ears. The neck is powerful and well set-on. Short body. Short, powerful, slightly sloping croup. Stable constitution with clean joints and broad hooves. The colour of the foals varies from dark brown through reddish brown to light brown; there are also some light grey foals. The pure white colour is not achieved until the age of 5–7 years. Height 135–145 cm.

Distribution: The main habitat is the Rhone delta in southern France, in particular between Montpellier to the west, Tarascon to the north and Fos to the east. There are some animals in other European countries. Isolated animals in North–Rhine/Westphalia.

Uses: In its native region it is used by the 'Gardiens' for herding cattle. It is particularly lively and adept at this activity. Good endurance, undemanding. Well adapted to the marshes and sparse vegetation of the region; in the summer it feeds mainly on reed shoots, and in the winter on the salty vegetation of the steppe. Eminently suitable for leisure riding owing to its gentle nature and small size.

Breed history: One of the oldest horse breeds in the world. Presumed to derive from cross-breeding various forms of horse. The horse of the Camargue was familiar to the Phoenicians; Caesar is also said to have fostered the breed. Napoleon equipped his army mainly with the Camargue; it proved to be a successful pack animal when the Suez Canal was being built. In recent decades, Berbers and Arabs have been crossed with it. It is now bred for a somewhat larger type better suited to the changed conditions of cattle farming.

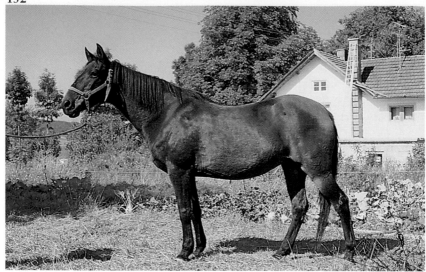

Berber

Characteristics: Small, clean, powerful horse. The long, powerful head is usually slightly convex. Broad chest, flat shoulders. Short back and steeply sloping croup. The tail is set low. Long legs with strong bones. All basic colours occur. Height 148–155 cm.

Distribution: North Africa. A few animals in other countries. Isolated examples are kept in the former West Germany and Switzerland.

Uses: Temperamental. Good-natured. Tough with good stamina. Frugal and willing.

Breed history: Berber horses were known in ancient times and were famed for their speed. It is assumed that the Berber also goes back essentially to coldbloods, which the Vandals brought with them from the north during the migratory era. When the Arabs came to North Africa in the seventh and eighth centuries, they brought their horses with them and crossed them with some of the native horse population. Horses with Berber blood then also came to Spain via the Arabs. As the Berbers with their rounded body shapes conformed best to the Baroque ideal of beauty, they came into the possession of many European rulers around this time, and thus started to be bred in those countries. In North Africa, larger, heavier horses were crossed with them by colonials. Many breeds all over the world have Berber ancestry, such as all American horse breeds introduced via Spain, the English Thoroughbred and the Lipizzaner.

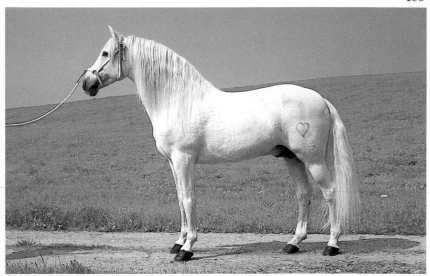

Andalusian

Characteristics: Refined, elegant horse, fairly deep and broad. Mostly grey with a blue sheen, but also black and other dark colours. Expressive head with straight or slightly convex profile. Curved, well set-on neck. Prominent withers. Correct shoulders. Elegantly carried tail. Very clean legs with short cannons and well-defined fetlocks. Height 155–160 cm.

Distribution: Spain. Significant holdings as well as isolated animals in the former Federal Republic of Germany and other European countries.

Uses: Agile and with good stamina. Free, smooth movements. High gait. Good jumper. Excellent for haute école. In Spain used for riding and as a coach horse as well as in bull fights.

Breed history: Descended from horses which the Phoenicians brought to Spain. Later, Berbers and Arabs were crossed with the indigenous horses by Muslim rulers. The breed had its golden age in the sixteenth and seventeenth centuries, when it had a great influence on almost all other European horse breeds. Lipizzaners and Kladrubers, in particular, are directly descended from Andalusians because, in Baroque times, the latter conformed most closely to the ideal of a beautiful horse. Only the monks of the Carthusian monastery at Jerez opposed a royal order to cross heavier horses and coldbloods with them. Thus the Andalusian survives to the present day. Several centuries ago they were also popular in central Europe, and they have been kept as a pure breed in the former West Germany for some years. Almost all Central and South American horses as well as the Western horses of North America can be traced back to the Andalusian.

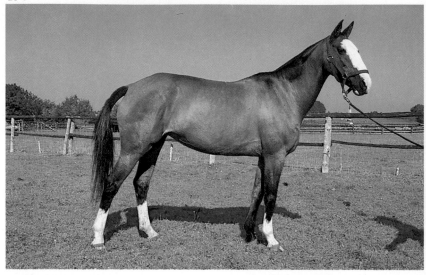

Argentinian Polo Pony

Characteristics: Refined, long-legged horse. Occurs in all basic colours, but brown predominates. The centre of the torso is short. Well-muscled. Height in general 150–160 cm. The term 'pony' is no longer really justified. It dates back to a time when polo ponies were considerably smaller.

Distribution: Spread from Argentina to all countries where polo is played. In recent years, numbers in the former Federal Republic of Germany have also increased.

Uses: Fast, agile and with good stamina. Has an astonishing ability to understand tasks and to grasp the rider's intentions. This applies not only to polo, but also to its use in cattle farming. It has 'cow sense'. Owing to this continual practice and the continuing selection of the most able animals, Argentinian Polo horses are prized all over the world.

Breed history: The game of polo was brought to the UK from India in 1870, and it soon spread from there to many other countries where equestrian sport was popular. Initially, indigenous ponies were used in these countries until, at the beginning of this century, Australian ponies were found to be the most suitable. From 1930 the Argentinian Polo Pony was so superior to other types of horse that it almost displaced them all over the world. This trend was intensified by World War II, when the sport of polo almost came to a halt, except in Argentina. Originally the Polo Pony was more a type for a specific purpose than a breed. For a long time only mares that have proved themselves in the sport have been used for breeding, so that the Polo Pony can be regarded as a true breed. The word polo is derived from the Tibetan word for ball – 'pulu'.

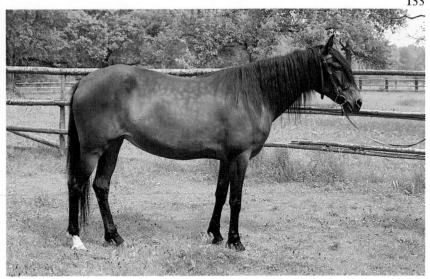

Peruvian Paso

Characteristics: It is said to radiate energy, strength, grace and vitality. It can be black, chestnut, grey, palomino, blue roan, or red roan. Dark nostrils. White markings allowed only on the lower legs, between the eyes and above the lips. Small, straight, finely shaped head. Broad forehead. Expressive eyes. Small muzzle. Large, thin-rimmed nostrils. Gracefully curving neck. The back is of short to medium length and strong. The chest is well-rounded and deep. The shoulders are rather sloping and well-muscled. The legs have well-defined tendons. Overall, the muscles are well-developed. Height 144–154cm.

Distribution: Peru, North America. Also central Europe in recent years.

Uses: Intelligent, obedient and always willing. The gait of the Paso is a broken pace, the pure four-beat toelt being greatly preferred. In the 'Termino' the front limbs are unfurled. It should travel down from the shoulder. This and other elements of the movement produce a free, fluid, rolling motion which gives rise to a smooth, elegant gait. A characteristic is that the rear hoof impression falls past the front hoof impression of the same side. Suitable for trekking and long-distance rides.

Breed history: Derived in Peru from the horses of the Conquistadors, essentially crossbreeds of Andalusians and Berbers. There the desire was for a hard, refined saddle horse with a smooth, comfortable gait, as owners of large estates were often in the saddle for 8–10 hours in order to cover the large distances on their extensive holdings.

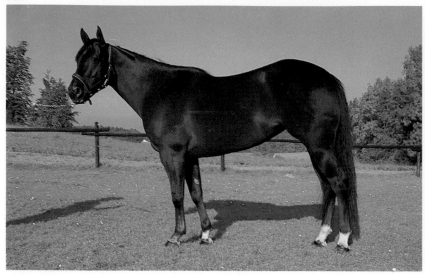

Quarter Horse

Characteristics: A compact horse with strong muscling. The most common colours are chestnuts and various shades of brown, but all colours and shades from grey to black are possible. Always mono-coloured with or without markings on the head and legs. Refined head. Short back. Powerful, sometimes top-heavy hindquarters. Height 145–156 cm, weight 520–680 kg.

Distribution: North and South America, Australia, central Europe and other regions.

Uses: Very versatile horse. It is the sprinter among horses. Superior to all other breeds over short distances. Invaluable assistance on ranches for driving and sorting cattle. In the USA it was used for races over a quarter of a mile, the ideal distance for it. This gave rise to its name. In North America it is used in Western shows and rodeos. Docile and easily trained.

Breed history: Developed at the beginning of the seventeenth century from horses of Spanish and English descent. It was recognised as a breed in 1665. Later, English Thoroughbreds were crossed with it. In the past it was used mainly on ranches. The first horse races in North America were held with the Quarter Horse, in Virginia. In 1941 the American Quarter Horse Association was founded. It has been kept in the former West Germany since the 1970s. By number of animals, it is the most common horse breed in the world.

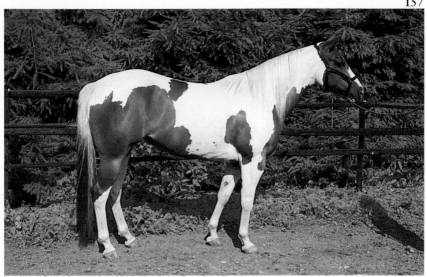

Paint

Characteristics: Compact, agile horse of medium size with well-developed muscling. Distinctly athletic. There are two different colour patterns. In the Overo, which is recessive, the white extends from the side, the belly or the legs. The white does not cross the back line. In the Tobiano, it appears to extend out from the back. The white markings cross the top line of the animal. Tobianos always have white legs. Small, wedge-shaped head. Alert eyes. Broad forehead. Small ears. Comparatively short neck. Shoulders well-muscled. Withers well-defined. The short back is well-knit to the hindquarters. The latter are very muscular, especially the powerful, sloping croup. Powerful constitution. Paints weigh 550–650 kg, and are 150–155 cm high.

Distribution: North America. Central Europe. UK. Japan. Australia. South Africa.

Uses: Robust and good-natured. Paints perform particularly well as short-distance race horses over a quarter of a mile. In North America they are used on ranches (cowboy horses) or as Western horses. The latter applies to a certain extent in Europe as well. They are good leisure and trekking horses.

Breed history: Part-coloured horses occurred from time to time among the Quarter Horse, and were excluded from breeding. Two groups of Paint breeders were formed, and they merged in 1965 to form the American Paint Horse Association. From the outset, this organisation recognised only horses of pure Quarter Horse descent as Paint Horses; it is therefore a part-coloured Quarter Horse.

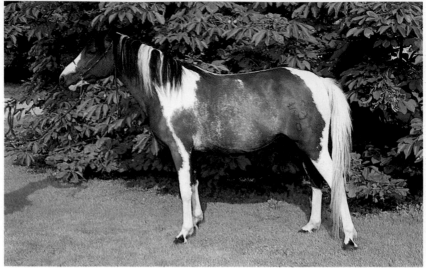

Pinto

Characteristics: Part-coloured Western horse of the 'Pleasure Type', i.e. a powerful, well-muscled horse, which is nevertheless elegant, with a refined head and a nicely curving neck. Short back. Long, sloping shoulders. Height 145–160 cm, weight 400–500 kg. The Pinto has the same two colour patterns as the Paint – Tobiano and Overo.

Distribution: Originally North America. Now also central Europe.

Uses: Fast, good stamina, undemanding. Used for Western shows as well as for long-distance riding, trekking and skill tests. Typical well-balanced horse that rides easily, has a friendly nature and intelligence. The original and typical Pinto also possesses 'cow sense' in working with cattle. First-class family and leisure horse.

Breed history: The same origins as the Paint Horse to some extent, but developed differently. Arabs were crossed with them over a period of time. There are four breed books with requirements of varying strictness:

- *Permanent Registration Division.* Any part-coloured horse of any breed may be registered.
- *Premium Registration Division.* At least one generation must be registered already.
- *Approved Breed Division.* Pure-bred Pintos, i.e. there are already several perfect Pinto offspring.
- *Solid Colour Breeding Stock Division.* Must be 100% inheritors of the colour, i.e. ancestors have been part-coloured for at least six generations.

A Pinto Horse Society was founded in 1941, but Pintos have only been officially recognised as a breed since 1963.

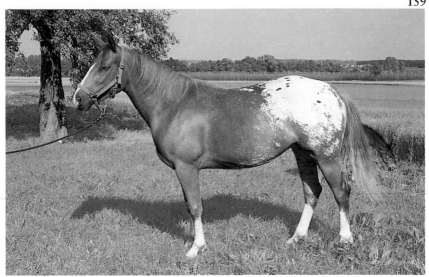

Appaloosa

Characteristics: Well-muscled, square-shaped horse. The most prominent feature is the partially spotted coat. Often the front half is fully pigmented (perhaps with markings), while the rear half of the body is white or white with spots of pigment. Often the entire coat is white with dark spots or spiky hairs. The base colour can vary from black through all shades of brown to golden yellow. There is often also a uniform mixture of red and white hairs, and greys can occur. Refined head. Straight nose line. Widely spaced eyes. The pupil has a white ring around it. Relatively short back. Deep body. Sloping croup. Fine hair in the mane and tail. Height 148–160 cm, weight 430–570 kg.

Distribution: North America, central Europe.

Uses: Tough. Hardy. Fast starter and sprinter, but also has stamina. Used for Western shows and racing. Suitable for leisure riding, and for children and young people. Owing to its placid temperament and its manageable size it is suitable for riding therapy.

Breed history: The Nez Percé Indians in the north west of the USA bred part-coloured horses from the start of the eighteenth century. White people first saw these horses by the little Palouse river which flows through this region. They designated them as 'a Palouse', which later became Appaloosa. The Indians selected their horses not only for their markings, but also for their speed and endurance. The Appaloosa was recognised as an independent breed in the USA in 1950. In recent decades, American Quarter Horses, Arabs and other breeds have been crossed with them occasionally.

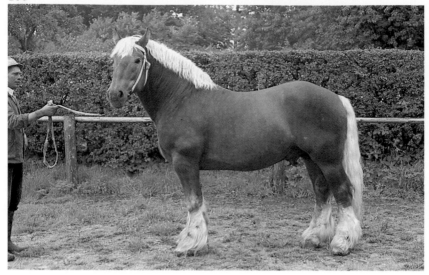

Schleswig Heavy Draught

Characteristics: Low, short-legged, compact horse of medium build. Predominantly chestnut; there are a small number of greys. The silky feather is typical. Height 156–162 cm, weight is about 800 kg.

Distribution: Schleswig–Holstein and Lower Saxony. Isolated numbers in other parts of the former Federal Republic of Germany.

Uses: Outstanding draught animal in agriculture, especially on heavy marshy ground. It was also used by hauliers and forestry operators in the past. Extensive stride and trotting gait. Lively but good-natured temperament. Good stamina, undemanding.

Breed history: The Schleswig Heavy Draught is descended from the Jutland horse of Denmark. The introduction of the stallion Oppenheim around 1860 was important for the Danish breed and hence also for the Schleswig Heavy Draught. Its precise origin is uncertain; it may have been Suffolk or Shire. In 1891 the Association of Schleswig Horse Breed Societies was founded. This breed had its golden age in the years following World War II, when the Association encompassed more than 15,000 breeders with about 20,000 brood mares. Later, attempts were made to modernise the breed by crossbreeding with stallions of the French Boulonnais. Some years ago, Jutland stallions and mares were bought to increase the build and to strengthen the constitution. Originally, the breeding centre was in the northern provinces of the state of Schleswig–Holstein. Now it is in the province of Segeberg. There are currently about 80 mares and 19 stallions in the stud book. The state of Schleswig–Holstein sponsors the preservation of the breed.

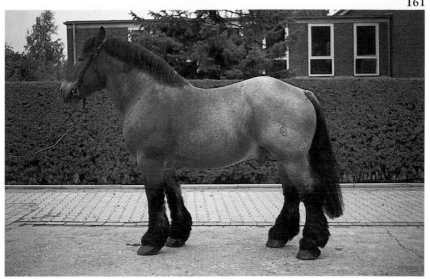

Rhineland–Westphalian Heavy Draught

Characteristics: Powerful working horse of broad build, medium weight and medium size. Mainly dappled grey; also chestnut and bay. Attractive head on a powerful neck. Compact, sloping shoulders. Deep, broad chest. Short, muscular back. Divided croup. Short limbs. Height 163–173 cm, weight up to 1000 kg.

Distribution: North-Rhine/Westphalia. Breeding pockets in Lower Saxony, Hesse and Rhineland–Palatinate. Isolated animals in other states of the former West Germany.

Uses: Powerful, robust, willing horse. Placid temperament. Occasionally it is still used in agriculture and increasingly in forestry. Currently, it is used by breweries, mainly for promotional purposes. Matures early. Frugal.

Breed history: Intensification of agriculture and industrialisation in the middle of the last century required a heavy commercial horse. English cold-bloods were used first, then later Belgian Heavy Draughts and Ardennes were preferred. These had influenced Rhenish horse breeding since the start of the nineteenth century. In 1892 the Rhenish horse stud book was founded. In the 1930s this breed constituted 50% of the total horse population of the German Empire. After World War II its commercial importance fell sharply. In 1957 the state stud at Wickrath, which had been founded in 1839, was dissolved; the remaining Heavy Draughts were transferred to the Westphalian state stud at Warendorf. In recent decades there has been considerable shrinkage, and the former heavy carthorse has become a medium-framed horse. The Westphalian horse stud book now contains about 400 mares and 46 stallions.

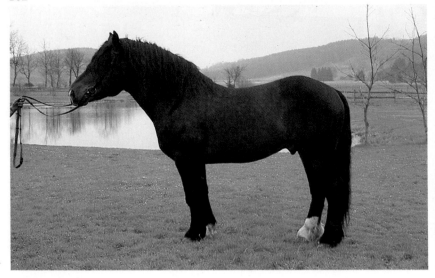

South-German Coldblood

Characteristics: Medium-sized, tough, very clean coldblood horse. Good fore-quarters. Fairly long but taut mid-quarters. Firm, broad loins. Long, divided croup. Well-muscled. Good depth and correct constitution. Mainly bay and chestnut. Height 155–165 cm, weight 700–900 kg.

Distribution: Baden–Württemberg, Bavaria.

Uses: Prolific, long-lived, frugal. Good character. Agile and versatile. Suitable for agricultural work and timber-hauling in the mountains and on flat land. Long stride. In recent years it has often been used as a coach horse in tourist areas and as a show horse in carnival processions.

Breed history: In centuries past, a coldblood horse was bred in Bavaria which was said to be descended from horses of the Roman province of Noricum, and was therefore called a Noriker. There were two types: the heavy strain was called 'Pinzgauer', and the light strain 'Oberländer'. Over a period of time, warmblood and cold-blood stallions of other breeds, both domestic and foreign, were often crossed with them. Later, attempts were made to reinforce the type and to make it homogeneous. Austrian stallions were then used. After World War II, the two strains were combined under the designation 'South German Coldblood'. The State Association of Bavarian Horse Breeders encompassed about 28,000 mares and 600 stallions of this breed after the war. There was no real decline in the breed until the 1960s. Currently it is not possible to meet the demand for this horse in Germany.

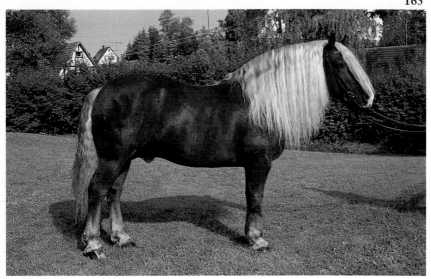

Black Forest Fox

Characteristics: Light to medium-weight, balanced coldblood horse. Fine head. Short, powerful and well set-on neck. Short midquarters. Broad croup. Powerful, clean constitution with little feather on the pasterns. Hard hooves. The colour is mostly dark brown, the long hair being light, often almost white (liver chestnut). Mares are 150 cm high, stallions several centimetres higher.

Distribution: The Black Forest area.

Uses: Good-natured, yet lively. Good draught animal with stamina. Agile and tough. Long, smooth gait. Used in forestry work and on smallholdings. Used in tourism as a coach and sleigh horse, but also suitable for leisure riding. Undemanding. Thrives even on the lime-free land of the upper Black Forest.

Breed history: There have been coldblood horses in the Black Forest for many hundreds of years. At first, all colours were found. The chestnuts can be traced back mainly to a stallion born in 1875. In 1896, breeders joined together to form the Black Forest Horse Breed Cooperative. Their animals were shown for the first time under the breed title Black Forest Horses at a DLG show in 1906. Up to the end of World War II, stallions of many different coldblood breeds, and also warmbloods, were used for cross-breeding. After the war, numbers fell at first; from 1970 the trend was upwards again. There are about 170 registered mares and ten stud stallions. In recent years the breed has become somewhat more disparate again with the purchase of Noriker stallions. Stallions are now reared and kept at the state stud at Marbach.

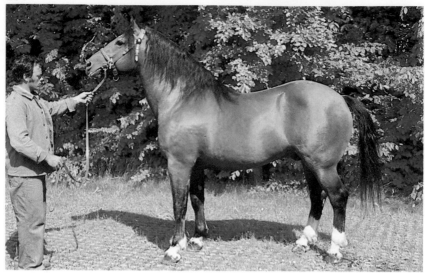

Freiberger

Characteristics: Powerful, but not heavy coldblood. Brown is the most common colour, but chestnut occurs quite frequently. Small, expressive head. Massive neck. Broad chest. Slightly rounded croup. Powerful, clean limbs. Short pasterns. Good hooves. Height 150–155 cm, weight 550–650 kg.

Distribution: Switzerland. Isolated animals in other countries, primarily for crossing with heavy coldblood breeds to give the latter a somewhat smaller frame.

Uses: Expressive, contented, obliging horse, matures early. Good character. Frugal. Correct, economical gait. The Freiberger is an ideal draught, pack and saddle horse for the purposes of agriculture in hilly areas. In Switzerland it is also still often used for military purposes and is invaluable in forest work.

Breed history: The original habitat of this horse is the Swiss Jura, especially the high plateau of the Freiberg, where it has been kept for centuries. During the nineteenth century, stallions of 10 different breeds were used, in particular Anglo–Norman and Belgian Coldblood, but also Thoroughbred. The breed has been consolidated since the start of this century. After World War II, the population fell to one-fifth of the earlier maximum of 80,000 animals. It has better prospects than other coldblood breeds owing to its lighter calibre and its use by the Swiss Army for pack duty in the mountains.

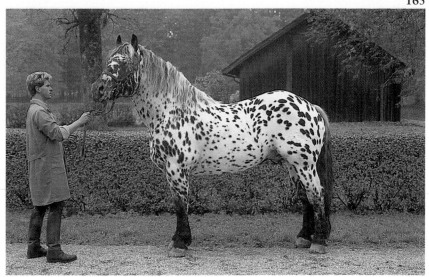

Noriker

Characteristics: Coldblood of medium build. They may be bay, chestnut, blue roan, spotted and, very rarely, they may have a black head. Large, heavy head. Short, powerful neck. Broad chest. Rather sloping shoulders. Long, broad back. Legs of medium length with well-formed hocks and little feather on the pasterns. Height about 160 cm.

Distribution: Austria, primarily the mountainous regions. The main breed range is around the Grossglockner. Exported to neighbouring countries and also to Pakistan and China.

Uses: Versatile commercial horse of outstanding ability. Good character with adequate temperament and refinement. Sure-footed.

Breed history: The Noriker is said to be descended from horses of the Roman Legion. It has been rigorously subjected to pure breeding and strict selection for over 400 years. In 1574 the first land studs were sent to Pinzgau by Archbishop Kuen. In 1688 Archbishop Count Thun stipulated the following rules, which had a decisive influence on Noriker breeding. 1. Native brood mares may only be served by native stallions. 2. Only Court stallions may be used for covering. 3. The state may only buy foals sired by Court stallions. During the Renaissance, Andalusian and Neapolitan stock was crossed with the native horse population. There are currently about 9,000 Norikers, of which 2,700 are registered as main stud book mares with the individual breed associations. Norikers are the only coldblood breed still kept in a closed breed range entirely on farms. Numbers have consolidated in recent years. In 1984 the first Federal Noriker Show for 18 years took place in Wels (Upper Austria).

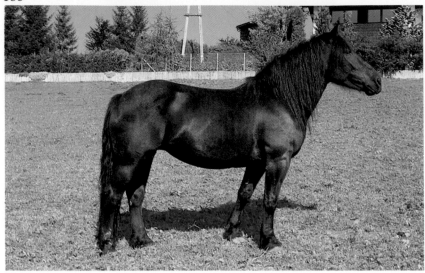

Abtenau

Characteristics: Smallest coldblood of the German-speaking countries. Classed as a special small form of the Noriker. Balanced build with refined head and powerful constitution. They are mainly black, but there are also various shades of chestnut. Animals with black heads are particularly distinctive: blue roans with black heads, which should have no forehead markings if possible. Unlike the Pinzgau, there are no spotted animals. The weight is variable, about 600 kg, height 148–154 cm. In recent years there has been a trend towards heavier animals of larger build.

Distribution: The Abtenau (centred on the village of the same name), a high valley south-east of Salzburg.

Uses: Undemanding, contented, robust horse. Agile and well suited to working on mountain slopes and hauling timber on small and medium-sized local farms. Energetic and willing. In the Austrian Federal Army, an infantryman who can march particularly well is said to 'walk like an Abtenau'. Distinctly well-balanced. Pacid temperament. Now often used as a carriage horse.

Breed history: It has been a separate form among the Noriker strains from time immemorial. Particularly small Noriker stallions are currently used as studs. There are about 70 brood mares.

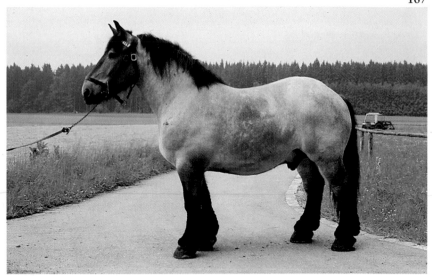

Belgian Coldblood

Characteristics: Heavy, powerful coldblood horse. Bay, chestnut, or various shades of grey (mainly brown roan). Small, expressive head on a short, heavy neck. The build is round; stocky and low slung. The body is well-proportioned. Well-knit mid-quarters. Broad chest and powerfully muscled croup. The legs are short and strong with a lot of feather. Stallions are on average 172 cm high and reach a weight of more than 1100 kg. Mares are somewhat lighter and smaller.

Distribution: It has become the most internationally widespread of all coldblood breeds. It is bred in many European countries as well as in North and South America. There are still a few examples in the former Federal Republic of Germany.

Uses: Outstanding workhorse. Enormous strength as a draught animal. Good-natured temperament. Easily controlled. Good trotter for its weight. Frugal. Matures early.

Breed history: Coldbloods have been bred in Belgium since time immemorial. Caesar praised a tough, tireless farm horse that lived to the west of the Rhine. The powerful and temperamental Belgian horse also enjoyed a good reputation in the Middle Ages. Heavy horses were also very popular in the Age of Chivalry. Later, agriculture required heavy, powerful horses. At the end of the nineteenth century, the various strains which had been separate until then were unified. Nevertheless, a distinction is still made between the larger and heavier Brabant and the smaller and lighter Ardennes.

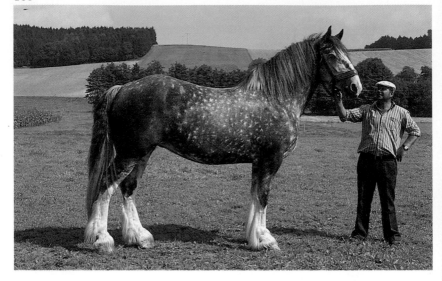

Shire

Characteristics: Largest breed of horse in the world. The colours are brown, black, chestnut and grey. Large white spots on the body are undesirable. Distinctive extensive white markings on the legs. Large, heavy head. Short, powerful, well set-on neck. Short, strong back. Long, broad, well-muscled croup. A characteristic feature is the extensive feather on the legs, which starts at the foreleg knee and hock and surrounds the pastern and hoof in long thick hair. Mares reach a height of 165–178 cm. A mature stallion is 170–180 cm high, and weighs 1000–1200 kg

Distribution: The UK, North and South America, South Africa and Australia.

Uses: Extraordinary strength. Healthy constitution. Hardy. Friendly, obliging. Fairly phlegmatic temperament. It is used as a draught animal for heavy loads: brewers' drays, timber wagons. In the UK it is also used for pro-

motional purposes.

Breed history: The Shire is a descendant of the warhorse of the Age of Chivalry. It comes from the shires of Leicestershire, Staffordshire and Derbyshire in the UK. Originally bred for military purposes, it was later used in agriculture as cultivation of the land intensified. The breed had to be developed to be suitably heavy, especially for working heavy marshlands. In 1878 the Shire Horse Society was founded in the UK, and now has more than 2,500 members. In the past, Shires were predominantly black, and were thus also called Old Black English Cart Horses.

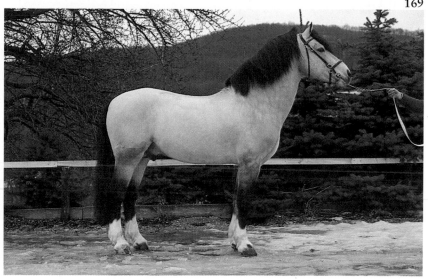

Welsh Cob

Characteristics: Medium-sized, compact, powerful horse, its conformation being between those of the warmblood and the coldblood. Refined, expressive, pony-like head. Broad forehead, lively eyes, small ears. Well set-on, powerful neck with a curving top line in the case of stallions. Powerfully muscled, sloping shoulders. Short back, well-sprung ribs, large girth. Well-muscled croup and hindquarters. Short legs. Strong cannons, clean pasterns. Hard hooves. Silky feather on pasterns. All colours occur. White markings are acceptable, but patches of colour are not. Height from 137 cm, but mostly between 148 and 155 cm. Animals reared on the continent of Europe are generally larger than those reared in Wales.

Distribution: UK. Central Europe. North America.

Uses: Hardy. Undemanding. Good endurance. Lively. Good-natured and placid. Outstanding walking ability.

Smooth, energetic action from the shoulder. Powerful thrust from the hindquarters. Considerable jumping ability. Excellent coach horse. Extremely agile. Crossing cobs and other breeds often produces distinctly well-balanced and able horses.

Breed history: The Welsh Cob is native to Wales. It can be traced back partly to Spanish horses, but at the time of the Roman invasion there were already small, powerful but nimble horses in Wales. In the last century, Arabs and English Thoroughbreds were crossed with it. This did not alter the type. In its mountain habitat the Cob has been used in agriculture for centuries, and has also been used as a carriage horse and for war duties. The first stud book was opened in 1902. Horses which do not achieve a height of 137 cm are entered as Welsh Ponies, Section C.

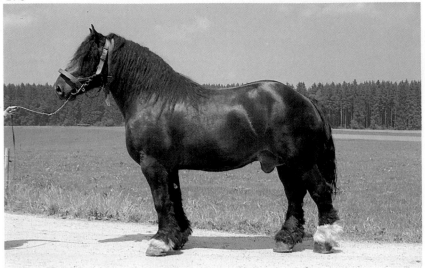

Percheron

Characteristics: Heavy coldblood. The colours are grey and black. Fine head with lively eyes and long, fine ears. Straight nose line. Large nostrils. Long, powerful neck. Distinctly sloping shoulders. Broad, deep chest; well-sprung ribs. Short, straight back. Deep girth. Long, slightly sloping, divided croup. Powerful, but clean limbs. A lot of feather on the pasterns. Well-muscled overall. Height 155–172 cm, weight on average 900 kg.

Distribution: Mainly north-west France, but also other areas of the country. Also found in the UK, the USA, Japan, and many other countries. Smaller numbers in the former Federal Republic of Germany.

Uses: Outstanding draught horse. Possesses great energy, endurance and willingness to work. Light, flexible stride; elegant trotter. Its temperament requires a firm hand. In the former Federal Republic of Germany it is used mainly by breweries and forestry operations. In France it is reared extensively for meat.

Breed history: The Percheron is native to the former province of Perche, now the départements of Orne and Eure et Loire. It is an ancient breed, with which Arabs were crossed in the eighth century. Later, Spanish, Norman and, repeatedly, Arab stallions contributed to the development of the breed. There were several strains for a long time. Only the heaviest survived, meeting the demands of agriculture and the needs of the main country of export, the USA.

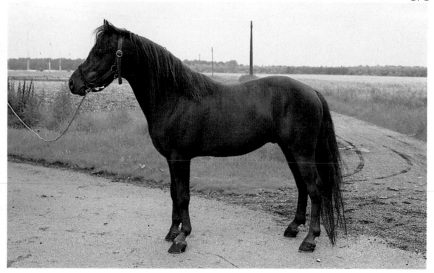

German Riding Pony

Characteristics: The name denotes a line of breeding, not a breed. It covers animals produced by crossing various pony breeds and also by crossing ponies with full-size horses. The following definition can be regarded as the breeding plan: a willing pony suitable for the saddle and harness for children and adults, with the proportions and movement of a saddle horse while maintaining the distinct type of the pony, such as a short, broad head with large eyes, good muscling with rounded contours, and a solid constitution; minimum height 138 cm (maximum 148 cm). Ideas on the standard to be aimed for have not yet been unified everywhere.

Distribution: The former Federal Republic of Germany, especially Westphalia.

Uses: Rides well and is willing. Obliging, has good stamina and is undemanding. It has no faults of temperament or character. Can be used for riding and in harness. Frugal.

Breed history: It has been developed from Dülmeners, Nordkirchners, as well as British and other pony breeds, and in recent decades from Arabs and other full-size horse breeds.

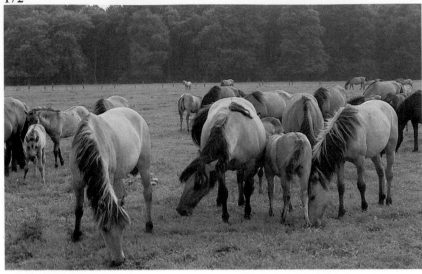

Dülmener

Characteristics: Primitive horses of all colours and shades, three colour strains being predominant: dark bay with a pale muzzle (similar to Exmoor Ponies); golden bay and dun (probably of Przewalski stock); mousy grey with a back line and a suggestion of stripes on the forelegs. They may also be chestnut, bay and grey. Long, dense mane and long tail. Small, very hard hooves. Height 125–135 cm.

Distribution: The main population of about 200 animals is kept in an area of about 200 hectares in the Merfeld fault near Dülmen in Westphalia. The animals live outdoors all year round and are only given roughage in the winter. On the last Saturday in May, the yearling males are separated from the herd and auctioned. Isolated animals are kept in Westphalia in agricultural enterprises, on small-holdings or as a hobby.

Uses: Tough. Robust. Resistant to harsh weather. The herd living in the wild is not used in any specific way. After appropriate training they can be harnessed to carriages and make an appealing picture.

Breed history: Reference was made to it in the fourteenth century. The Dülmener, contrary to what one may read occasionally, is not a wild horse but is thoroughly domesticated. Apparently it was originally the result of cross-breeding between escaped domestic horses and wild horses. Later, stallions of several very disparate European breeds of primitive horses were used for breeding, in particular from Poland and the UK. Currently, its own stallions are used for breeding.

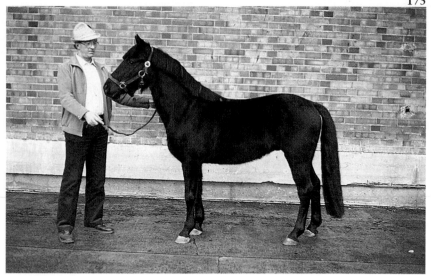

Nordkirchner

Characteristics : Light pony. They may be black, bay, chestnut and occasionally grey. Height 132–140 cm.

Distribution: Westphalia. Occasionally occurs in other states of the former Federal Republic of Germany, and in neighbouring countries.

Uses: Robust and hardy. Temperamental and willing to work. Also suitable as a saddle and carriage horse.

Breed history: Developed after World War I by crossing Panje horses with Dülmeners. Later Arabs and finally Welsh (Section B) were crossed with them. This made them larger, lighter and more like a riding pony than the Dülmener. At the Nordkirchner Rehbusch Forest Lodge there are now only remnants. Offspring produced by crossing with Arabs are much in demand in Germany and abroad. The Nordkirchner has largely been absorbed into the breeding of riding ponies in Westphalia.

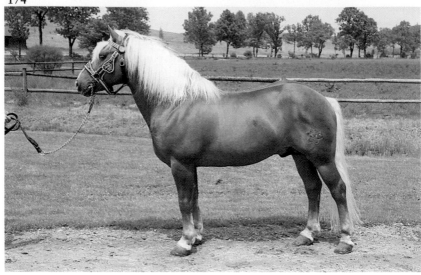

Haflinger

Characteristics: Small, stocky, well-balanced horse with fine long lines and good muscling. Chestnut, ranging from pale, golden light chestnut to dark liver chestnut. Clean, hard bones. Small head with lively, clear eyes and small ears, indicating Arab influence. Good hooves. Thick mane, preferably flaxen colour. Powerful, slightly wavy tail. Markings are common. Height 135–145 cm, weight 350–400 kg.

Distribution: Austria, Italy, the former Federal Republic of Germany, Switzerland and about 20 other countries. In Germany they are concentrated in Bavaria and Westphalia.

Uses: Excellent multi-purpose horse for agriculture and work with mountain troops. Sure-footed, good stamina. Outstanding climber. Good leisure horse for children and adults. Very good-natured and willing.

Breed history: In Roman times there were small pack horses in South Tyrol, and these are regarded as the ancestors of the Haflinger. Later there was considerable cross-breeding with Norikers and Arabs. Since the turn of the century they have been called after the village of Hafling above Meran. The progenitor is considered to be the light bay crossbred stallion 'Folie', sired by an Arab stallion and born in 1874.

Initially kept only in South Tyrol for agriculture and as a pack horse for mountain troops. After World War I, holdings were built up in Austria, and in the 1930s in Bavaria.

Modification of the uses to which the breed was put has altered the type in recent decades. Instead of the short-legged, small, coldblood, the demand is now rather for a small riding horse with a long neck, prominent withers and a correct, fluid gait. This is achieved by strict selection and by cross-breeding with Arabs.

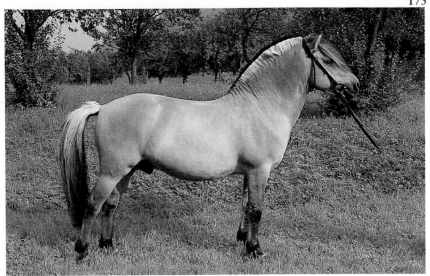

Fjord

Characteristics: Robust small horse. Mostly dun with a black back line, which continues as a black line in the mane to the ears and as a black band in the tail. There is often a hint of zebra striping on the legs. Small white markings on the head are allowed, but not on the legs. Large, nicely shaped head with broad forehead, large eyes and a straight or slightly concave nose line. Short ears. Short, powerful neck which merges into the normally long back with almost no withers. Sloping, well-muscled shoulders. Deep girth. Long forearm and short mid-foot. Pasterns fairly long. Croup short, pointed and sloping. Height 135–145 cm, weight 350–500 kg.

Distribution: Norway. All other parts of northern and central Europe. In the former West Germany they are concentrated in Hesse.

Uses: Suited to forestry work, part-time businesses and special businesses such as fruit-growing and viticulture. Suitable as a leisure horse, even for heavy adults. Lively, long, nimble gait with power and thrust from the hindquarters. Good-natured. Willing and obliging. Robust and frugal.

Breed history: Old Norwegian breed. It was developed in extensive husbandry in the harsh climate of the north, without the introduction of outside stock. In Norway it is used in agriculture. Introduced into Germany in the 1950s for the same purpose. As increasing mechanisation reduced agriculture's need for them, and the demand for riding ponies increased, the breeding plan changed from the broad, deep commercial conformation to the more refined, cleaner type with good withers and good walking ability.

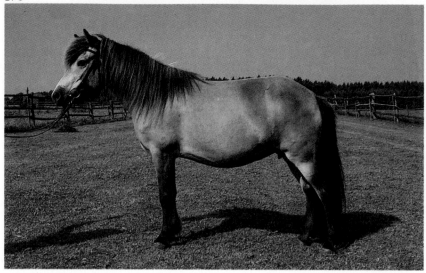

Icelandic Pony

Characteristics: Stocky, compact riding pony. Chestnut, black or bay, less commonly grey or part-coloured. Short, broad, fairly light head with small ears and a bushy forelock. Short neck with powerful mane. The shoulders are long, sloping and well-muscled. Powerful, tough build. Divided, slightly raised, sloping croup. Short, strong legs. Often splay-footed. Short, powerful pasterns. Hard, durable hooves. Coarse coat which repels rain well. The desired height is 130–138 cm with a weight of 350–400 kg.

Distribution: Iceland. Many countries in continental Europe. In the former Federal Republic of Germany it is concentrated in Rhineland and Palatinate.

Uses: Originally used as a draught horse in agriculture and for travel. Bred as a saddle animal for use in the rough country in its native land. Very sure-footed. In addition to the three common gaits it uses the tilt and pace.

Robust riding pony. Suitable for adults. Placid temperament. Tough and frugal. May be reared extensively with shelter.

Breed history: In the ninth and tenth centuries, the Vikings brought Scandinavian and Celtic ponies to Iceland. Since then the Icelandic Pony has had no introduction of outside stock in its own country. At about the turn of the century planned breeding was started. First exported to Germany in fairly small numbers in the 1930s. Greater numbers exported from the 1960s.

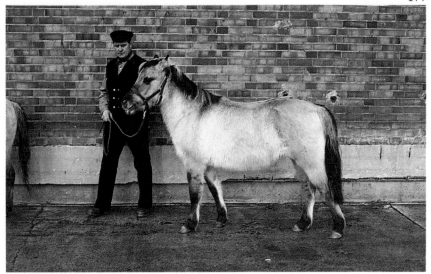

New Tarpan

Characteristics: Stock, muscular pony. Mousy grey to blue-grey. Light, short head. Broad forehead. Large eyes. Fine constitution. The mane has a slight tendency to be upright. There is often a suggestion of zebra striping on the legs. Stallions are 120–130 cm high and weigh 300–350 kg. Mares are on average 5 cm lower and 50 kg lighter.

Distribution: In the former West Germany it is kept in East Friesland and in some animal parks. Most animals are kept in Poland and the former Soviet Union.

Uses: Very prolific. Good mothers. Well-developed herd instinct. Good-natured.

Breed history: Wild or feral horses that were quite common in the Ukraine in the seventeenth century were called Tarpans. Wild horses lived in north-east Poland and in Lithuania into the eighteenth century. The latter were caught and kept in captivity. At the start of the nineteenth century the herds were disbanded and the horses were distributed among local farmers. They were absorbed into the Koniks, the local landrace. After World War I, 17 animals that were suitable in appearance and size were collected together in Poland, and a breed was developed from them. Now, several herds are kept there in conditions resembling the wild. In Germany, attempts were made to breed them in the 1930s in Hellabrunn in Munich. The horses used were Icelandic and Gotland mares mated with a Przewalski stallion. Since the start of the 1970s there has been a herd at Wittmund in East Friesland, which is descended from the Polish stock. Appropriate selection for breeding means that the new form closely resembles the earlier wild form.

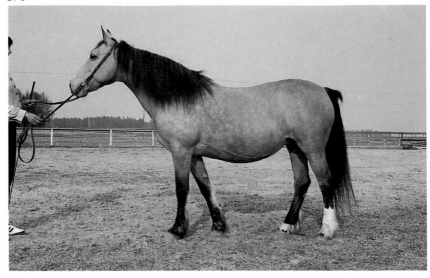

Connemara Pony

Characteristics: Well-balanced, compact, refined riding pony. All colours occur. Until a few decades ago, the dun colour was most common, as a result of the Andalusian/Spanish blood. As Arab stallions have been introduced from time to time, grey is now the dominant colour. Refined, fairly large head with relatively large ears. Long, well set-on, not over-developed neck. Long, sloping shoulders. Well-defined withers. Straight, strong back. Long, slightly sloping croup; well-muscled, becoming feathered lower down. Deep girth. Powerful, clean limbs. Well-formed, hard hooves. Height 142–148 cm. In size they are ponies, but in conformation they are small horses.

Distribution: Originally Ireland, now almost world-wide. They are concentrated in the UK and France, and are becoming more popular in Bavaria.

Uses: Good, long stride and galloping ability and an excellent jumper. Combines the riding characteristics of a full-sized horse with the hardiness and frugality of a pony. Agile and surefooted. Placid nature. Well-balanced temperament.

Breed history: Connemara in the province of Connaught in the west of Ireland has been the home of this pony for centuries. Descended from horses of the Exmoor type. In the nineteenth century and early twentieth century, coldbloods, Arabs, and English Thoroughbreds were introduced to give more calibre and commercial suitability to these horses which had been used primarily as riding ponies until then. There has been a breeding programme since 1923 when the Irish Pony Breed Society was founded. After that, Thoroughbred stallions were used. Since 1951 no stallions of other breeds have been used. Connemaras first came to the Continent at the start of the 1960s. The stud book in Ireland contains about 3000 mares and 200 stallions.

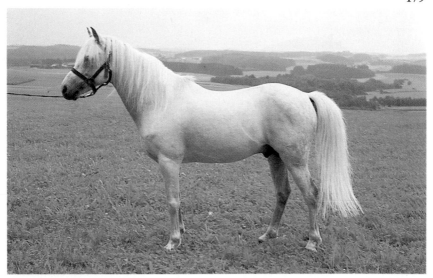

New Forest Pony

Characteristics: Refined, tough pony, which is not uniform in type. All colours apart from part-coloured are allowed. The basic colours are all shades of brown and chestnut. The original conformation has a medium-sized, clean head and a short neck. Fairly long back. Steeply sloping shoulders. High withers. Deep chest. Powerful renal region. Croup often sloping. High-set tail. Good constitution. The refined animals are 138–148 cm high; the semi-wild ones are about 10 cm lower.

Distribution: The New Forest area in the south of England, and the Netherlands. In the former Federal Republic of Germany they are concentrated in Schleswig–Holstein, Lower Saxony and Bavaria.

Uses: Placid temperament. Suitable as a riding horse for both children and adults. Can gallop and jump well.

Breed history: In the tenth century reference was made to small horses existing in the current area of distribution of this breed in the south of England. Up to 1938, many breeds were crossed with the ancient type. No outside stock has been used for about the last 30 years. About 3,000 animals are allowed to range freely, and receive no feed or shelter even in winter. There are also numerous studs which breed an improved, larger form by using Thoroughbreds. Many New Forest ponies were exported to the former Federal Republic of Germany in the 1970s.

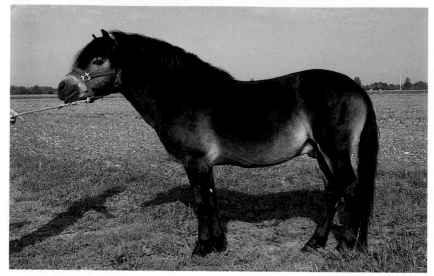

Exmoor Pony

Characteristics: Stocky, well-balanced build. They may be bay, dark bay or dark dun. Black nostrils. Mealy muzzle. Lighter on the belly, the inside of the front and rear thighs, and around the eyes. Broad forehead. Slightly protruding eyes. Short, thick, pointed ears. Wide nostrils. Deep, broad chest. Medium-length back with strong loins. The tail falls close to the rear legs. The shoulders are well set back and make it sure-footed. Clean legs with very hard hooves. Height 114–130 cm.

Distribution: UK. Various countries of continental Europe and North America. Only a few examples in the former West Germany.

Uses: Extremely tough and hardy. Good stamina, agile and very responsive.

Breed history: Represents a very ancient type of horse. It has lived on Exmoor, a wild area in the south-west of England, for centuries. It is popular for crossing with other breeds. The introduction of other breeds has not proved to be worthwhile.

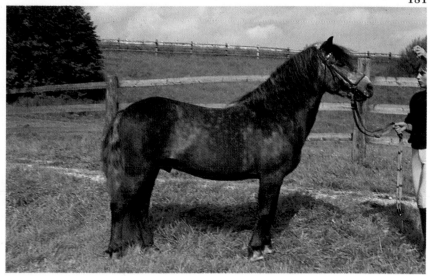

Dartmoor Pony

Characteristics: Refined and elegant. Predominantly bay or black, but all colours are allowed, except piebald and skewbald. Small, fine head. Small ears. Long, nicely arched, fairly light neck. The back, renal area and hips are powerful and muscular. Good saddle position. Croup short and sloping, with high set-on tail. Fairly strong legs. Very hard and well-formed hooves. A height of 120–127 cm is desirable.

Distribution: Mainly the county of Devon in the south-west of England. In the former Federal Republic of Germany there are breeding pockets in Schleswig–Holstein and Bavaria.

Uses: Very popular riding horse for children, with a good stride, can trot and gallop well, excellent jumper. Placid and reliable.

Breed history: It has lived for centuries on the heaths and moors of Dartmoor in the south-west of England. At the end of the nineteenth century the

Dartmoor type was established and a stud book was opened.

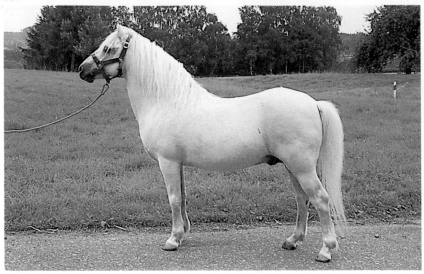

Welsh Pony

Characteristics: The Welsh Pony is bred in five strains, Sections A (**182**) to D differing essentially in size (Section A: maximum height 122 cm; Section D: a distinct element of full-size horse). The fifth strain, the Welsh Part-Bred, is the result of crossing Welsh Ponies of all Sections with other breeds. Originally the basic colours were bay and black. The Arab influence now means that grey is quite common. All colours are permitted, except piebald, skewbald and spotted. The following description applies to all except the Welsh Part-Bred: clean, fine head; large, clear, lively eyes. Small ears. Long, well set-on neck. Gently curved topline with naturally arching neck. Fairly high withers. Round croup, not too short, with high set-on tail. Long, sloping shoulders. Fairly heavy, clean constitution. Small firm hooves.

Distribution: UK. Central Europe. In the former West Germany, in Lower Saxony and Westphalia.

Uses: Depending on suitability and size, used for riding and light draught in the army and in agriculture, as well as a pack and pit horse. Good jumper or light draught horse, depending on Section. Its strength, endurance and walking ability make it a suitable progression for older children for leisure riding and arena events. Fluid, energetic movements; well-rounded action with a powerful thrust from the hindquarters.

Breed history: Animals in Section A are regarded as the original type. For more than 1000 years they have lived in the sparsely populated mountains of Wales. For more than 200 years, Thoroughbreds, Hackneys and Norfolk Trotters have been introduced into Section D from time to time (cf. Welsh Cob).

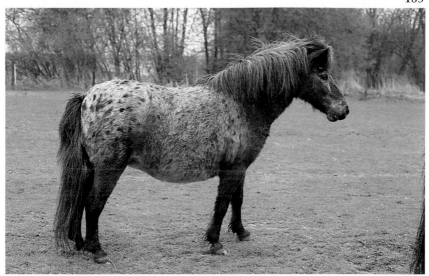

Shetland Pony

Characteristics: A dwarf horse which is obliging, refined, placid and intelligent. The basic colour is black; they may also be bay, chestnut, grey, part-coloured or (rarely) spotted. Clean, well-proportioned head with small, well set-on ears. Large, friendly eyes. Broad forehead, straight nose line, large nostrils. The neck is strong, muscular and short. Broad back. Well-muscled, fairly long croup. Tail set-on low. Sloping shoulders. Powerful legs. Hard, well-formed hooves. The coat varies depending on season: in summer it is short, smooth and shiny; in winter it is long, dense and firm. Thick mane, large forelock, long, thick tail. Height 98-106 cm (maximum), weight 150–200 kg.

Distribution: Mainly the region of origin, the Shetland Islands. Distributed almost world-wide. In the former Federal Republic of Germany, in Schleswig–Holstein and Lower Saxony.

Uses: From time immemorial, these tough, robust horses have been kept as pack and draught animals in their native habitat. They were used as pit ponies in coal mines in the UK. Their small size and good nature make them good riding horses for children. Their fast, clipped gait makes smooth riding difficult, however, especially at a trot. Can gallop and jump well. Good carriage horse for small carts. Good-natured, friendly and not easily startled. Easy to feed and care for.

Breed history: They have been kept for about 2000 years on the Shetland Islands. After the turn of the century they were brought to continental Europe by the Hagenbeck zoo in Hamburg. They achieved more widespread distribution there in later years. In North America they have undergone further development (cf. American Shetty).

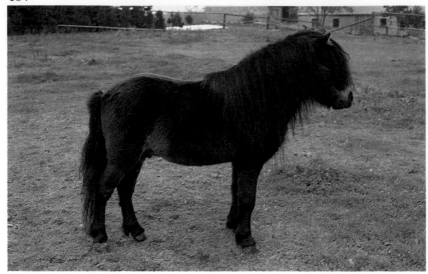

American Shetty

Characteristics: Small pony with proportions similar to those of a full-size horse. May be all one colour or part-coloured; all colours occur. Refined head, often pointed. Small ears. Slim midquarters. Slim legs, in proportion with respect to the body. Height up to 110 cm.

Distribution: North America. Central Europe.

Uses: Children's pony. Good-natured. Strong enough to pull twice its own weight and to carry up to 60 kg. Friendly nature. Adaptable. Easily trained.

Breed history: Was developed from the compact island conformation of the Shetland Pony. It is considerably more dainty and relatively longer-legged than the initial form. Shetland Ponies of this type are sometimes used on race tracks with tiny Sulkies in the USA. Mini-Shetties are not a separate breed. They are the smallest individuals of the American Shetland Pony, and are entered in a different register from the latter if they are below a height of 34 inches (86.4 cm). Enormous sums are paid for some animals: the smaller the horse, the higher the price. A price of $10,000 is quite possible for a fully grown animal which is less than 75 cm at the withers. References to miniature horses date back 300 years. Systematic breeding started around 1860. The small body size is often a result of depressive inbreeding. Apparently, Falabellas were introduced from time to time.

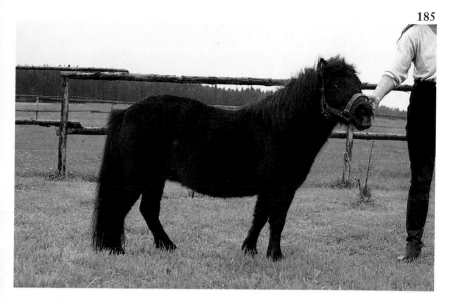

Falabella, Argentinian Dwarf Pony

Characteristics: Smallest horse breed in the world. They may be black, brown or grey. The average height is 65 cm, but some fully grown animals reach only 40 cm and weigh only 12 kg. Foals weigh 1–4 kg at birth.

Distribution: Argentina, North America, central Europe.

Uses: Garden or house horse. Occasionally they are used as a special attraction in the circus or zoo. Not suitable for the saddle or harness. The smaller they are, the more they cost.

Breed history: The breeding base consisted mainly of small Shetland Ponies, but also some larger horses. This breed is thought to have originated in a herd which was isolated in a ravine in the Andes of Argentina by a landslide. The animals remained cut off for generations and had very sparse fodder. This caused selection for small individuals. Julio Falabella discovered them there and rescued them from the ravine. Planned breeding began in 1868. The main stud is near Buenos Aires. The population now numbers about 1000 horses. Apparently, stallions are only rarely allowed to leave Argentina.

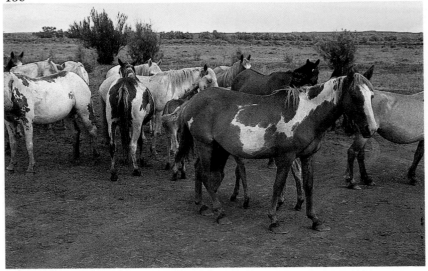

Mustang

Characteristics: Small, compact horse. All colours occur. Part-coloured animals are common. They have a large head, long ears, and a straight nose line. Clean limbs. Hard, flat hooves. Height 130–145 cm. Mustangs weigh about 450 kg (stallions), or 350 kg (mares).

Distribution: The west of the USA (mainly Nevada, Wyoming and Oregon), and of Canada. There are feral horses on some of the islands off the Atlantic coast of these countries. These have a different origin, however, and are designated differently.

Uses: Contented. Tough. Easily tamed.

Breed history: The word mustang is derived from the Spanish word *mestano*. It means that the animal does not belong to an individual person, but is common property. Mustangs are feral; i.e. they have no owner. Originally, the expression was used only for feral horses of Spanish descent; that is, for the animals and their offspring that escaped from the Spanish in the first phase of the settlement of North America, and became feral. At the end of the eighteenth and beginning of the nineteenth centuries it is estimated that there were 2–5 million feral horses in the area of today's USA. These were 120–130 cm high at the withers. At the beginning of the twentieth century, their size and weight increased, especially in their northern range, as they interbred with escaped or released warm-and-coldbloods of disparate ancestry. Mustangs formed the basis of a number of North American horse breeds. Before the Wild Free-Roaming Horse and Burro Act came into force in 1971, large numbers were culled and processed into animal feed. Excess animals are now captured and sold to enthusiasts for a few hundred dollars.

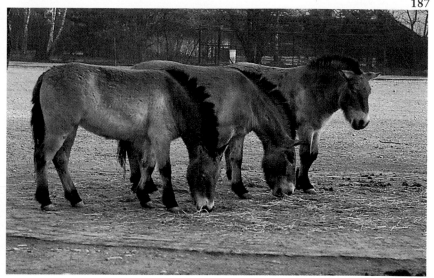

Przewalski's Horse

Characteristics: Stocky, compact wild horse with the conformation of a pony. The colour varies from dun with a hint of grey through reddish yellow to a strong red tone. The mane, tail and legs are black, and the area around the muzzle is almost white (mealy muzzle). It has a dark back line, a clear shoulder line, and sometimes zebra striping on the legs. Heavy head. Short ears (mouse ears). The upright mane is a notable feature. Height 130–155 cm. It has 66 chromosomes, unlike the domestic horse which has 64.

Distribution: There are almost 700 examples in zoos and reserves. It appears to be extinct in the region of origin of the type in Mongolia, near the Chinese border (in the Gobi desert between the Altai and Tienshan mountains).

Uses: Wild form. In captivity it has only exhibition value.

Breed history: According to cave paintings, it also lived in western Europe in the Palaeolithic age. It was presumably driven out into inhospitable regions by intense human persecution (competition with domestic animals for fodder, unwanted mating with domestic mares). In 1870 it was discovered in Mongolia by the Russian asiatic researcher Przewalski. In 1899 and 1902 a total of 58 horses were captured, only 11 of which are represented in recent blood lines. In 1947 another mare was captured, and there was also a Mongolian domestic horse mare. Today's Przewalski Horse population therefore is descended from 13 ancestors. Only 31 Przewalski Horses survived World War II. To preserve the type, an international stud book is kept in Prague, in which every individual is registered. In 1987, five animals from the Hellabrunn animal reserve in Munich were taken to a new breeding station in north-west China. The offspring will be released into the wild.

Donkeys and Mules

Only six species of the family of solid-hoofed ungulates (*Equidae*) have survived to the present day. The three zebra species and the half–donkey were apparently never domesticated, although it is occasionally assumed that the latter were. Only the horse and the donkey became domestic animals. All species can interbreed, but the offspring are almost always sterile. Mules are the result of crossing a female horse with a male donkey. A hinny results from crossing a female donkey with a male horse. Mules and hinnies differ in appearance: they always resemble the mother more than the father. In general, hinnies are smaller and lighter than mules. This is because, in addition to the reason given above, when mating female donkeys, which are smaller than female horses, male horses which are not much bigger are chosen to serve them. A full–size female horse, however, would be served by as large a male donkey as possible. Mules are produced more frequently than hinnies for the following reasons:

- It is easier to keep *one* donkey, namely a male, than *many* females.
- Male donkeys accept mares of the other species more easily as mating partners than do male horses.
- Owners prefer animals that resemble horses rather than donkeys.

Male mules and hinnies are always sterile, because sperm do not mature in their testes. Female animals of both types may occasionally be fertile, particularly if they have been covered by stallions of their mother's species.

Wild donkeys (*Equus africanus*) now only range freely in north–east Africa. There are two distinct forms: the Nubian Wild Donkey and the Somali Wild Donkey. It is assumed from archaeological finds that the donkey was domesticated in the Nile valley by 4000 BC (Hemmer, 1983). In central Europe the donkey was used mainly as a pack animal, while in other parts of the world it was used also as a draught animal. Here, it apparently played such an insignificant part in agriculture that it was scarcely mentioned in old veterinary science works and livestock breeding books. Presumably there was no breed selection; i.e. for uniformity in size, coloration or ability. There are only a few areas of the world where there was selection for particularly large or small donkeys, possibly because they were required for certain types of work, or because the conditions and available feed did not allow large animals to be kept. In central Europe there was in general great variety in donkey breeds, as there used to be among cattle and pigs until about 1850, among sheep until 1900 and among goats until 1930. In Germany, the advent of

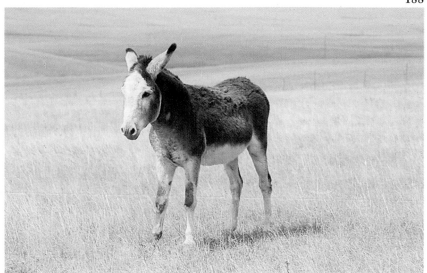

188 Feral donkey.

mechanisation heralded the decline of donkey breeding. Donkeys have always only been successful where they did not have to compete with motor vehicles, and where they were superior to horses in that they were cheaper, less demanding, or had greater ability in special situations. Today they occur primarily in the tropics and sub–tropics. In the second half of the last century in Germany asses' milk was used for dietary purposes, as it is an albumin milk, like human milk, while cows' milk is not. In some countries, special products were made from donkey meat in the past.

There is still a large donkey population in Switzerland, especially in Valais. Male donkeys are still used, but they are only bred to a limited extent; most of the animals come from Italy. In central Europe, mules also are used so infrequently that it does not justify the keeping of donkeys. When males are required for breeding they are usually brought from the Mediterranean region, where they are still largely irreplaceable. There are feral donkeys in many parts of the world (**188**). One reason is that they can survive well in inhospitable areas that cannot be used for agriculture. There they can easily become a threat to the indigenous fauna in competition for food. As the donkeys are more willing to approach water troughs, because they are less fearful of man, wild animals can be put at a dangerous disadvantage in time of drought. If they are not hunted, and are fed by man instead, feral donkeys soon become tame again. They may then become quite importunate.

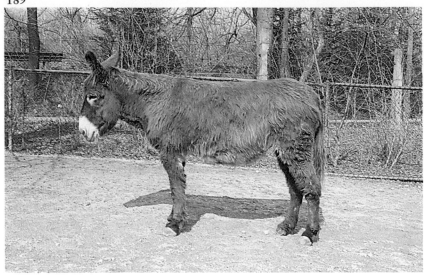

Poitou Donkey

Characteristics: Largest breed of donkey in the world. The coat is normally chestnut to dark brown, sometimes yellowish. The muzzle, nose and ears are silver-grey and have a reddish band around them. The underside of the belly and the insides of the thighs are pale. The hair is long and shaggy or almost curly. A notable feature is the particularly thick covering of hair on the large ears. The mane flicks from side to side. No back line. Heavy, bony head. Powerful neck. Straight shoulders. Long, straight back. Well-knit loins. Short croup. Haunches not very prominent. Long, muscular legs. Pasterns have long hair.

	Male	*Female*
Height at withers	145–155	140–150
Weight	350	300

Distribution: Originally bred over large areas of western France. Now it is kept only in the region of Melle in the Deux-Sèvres.

Uses: It is rarely used for work. Its main use is to produce mules, almost exclusively with mares of the 'Race Poitevine Mulassière'. Its meat is considered to be very good.

Breed history: According to records the Poitou Donkey has existed since the tenth century. It was often used to improve indigenous breeds of donkey in other Mediterranean countries and was exported to the USA. Although there has been a demand for Poitou Donkeys and the mules they produce in other countries, their numbers have declined since 1950. Recently, measures have been taken to preserve the breed by the French Agriculture Ministry in conjunction with the breeders and a regional wildlife organisation.

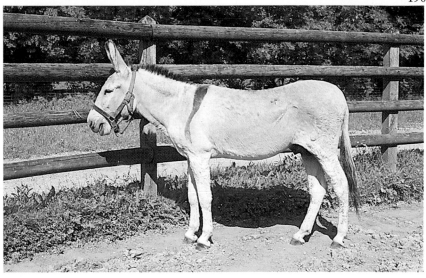

Donkey, medium-sized

Characteristics: All colours from white through grey (with and without some brown) to dark brown. Part-coloured animals are rare. Relatively heavy head, long ears and a broad muzzle. Large, rounded, prominent cheeks. Upright mane. Withers not prominent. Narrow chest, sloping croup. The tail has short hairs at the top and ends in a brush. The hooves have hard sides. Typically it has a dark lineback and a stripe extending down from it over the shoulders (shoulder cross). As there are no breeder organisations or breed standards, donkeys vary greatly in size, conformation and appearance.

	Male	Female
Height at withers	120–130	110–120
Weight	250–300	200–250

Distribution: Almost world-wide. In the former Federal Republic of Germany there are currently several hundred donkeys, of which nearly half are medium-sized animals.

Uses: Undemanding, patient animals with a friendly nature. Willing and tough. Contented. The meat is used for specialities, e.g. salami.

Breed history: Medium-sized donkeys were used in agriculture in central Europe for centuries. They were used for carrying loads (millers' donkeys) even into the twentieth century. The best known was the Thuringian Forest Donkey. The last examples of this breed are in the Erfurt zoo-park. They have been almost completely displaced by increasing affluence and mechanisation. Donkeys are feral in many countries (e.g. the USA, South America, Australia) and have become a threat to indigenous animals.

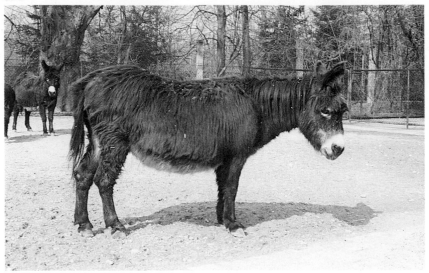

Dwarf Donkey

Characteristics: Well-proportioned animals with long ears, a sloping croup and dainty hooves. The colour varies from white through grey to black. They may also be part-coloured. The hair is of medium length; when they are kept in extensive conditions in the winter it forms a dense coat which determines the appearance of the animals.

	Male	Female
Height at withers	100–110	90–100
Weight	180–230	150–200

Distribution: Many Mediterranean islands (Sardinia, Sicily, Malta, Cyprus and islands in the Aegean Sea) and Sri Lanka. In recent times it has also been widely distributed in central Europe.
Uses: Patient, tough, good-natured animals, which are often expected to do amazing tasks in their countries of origin (pack, saddle and draught animals). In central Europe they are kept mainly by enthusiasts and as playmates for children.
Breed history: Dwarf Donkeys developed a very long time ago in various parts of the world. They are partly typical small forms, which often occur in other species as well on islands, and partly stunted forms which were the only ones to survive and reproduce in poor conditions and with sparse fodder. The animals kept on the only donkey breeding farm in the former Federal Republic of Germany are Dwarf Donkeys.

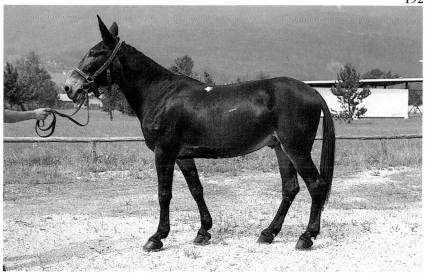

Mule

Characteristics: All characteristics are intermediate between those of the horse and the donkey. The colour varies from white to almost black; chestnut is very common. In comparison with a horse it has longer ears, a larger muzzle, a sparser mane, a thin tail and clumsy hooves. Its voice is between that of a horse and a donkey. The size is dependent on its parents, so all forms from dwarf to giant are possible.

Distribution: All countries where there are both horses and donkeys. Some countries import mules for specific purposes (e.g. the former Federal Republic of Germany). Other countries (e.g. Switzerland) import male donkeys from the Mediterranean area to produce mules.

Uses: Contented and with good stamina. Hardy. Patient. Long-lived. They have many of the positive characteristics of both the horse and the donkey. Sure-footed. In the mountains, hinnies carry loads of up to 130 kg, in addition to a saddle weighing almost 50 kg. They are generally sterile.

Breed history: In Switzerland, Italian male donkeys are used. The mules are used by the armed forces and in agriculture (mainly in the canton of Valais). In the former Federal Republic of Germany, the Bundeswehr in Bad Reichenhall has the last 'Mountain Pack-Animal Company', which uses mules. The animals are bought in Sicily. They must always be bred from the same initial species.

Pigs

Until quite recently it was thought that the domestic pig derived from two wild forms. Today it is agreed that only one species can be considered to be its ancestor: the wild pig (*Sus scrofa*). The earlier error is understandable. The wild form populates an enormous area, the north boundary of which lies between latitude 50 and 55 degrees and which extends from western Europe to eastern Siberia. In the south the range extends to India and south of the equator to the Indonesian archipelago. Within this area there are three sub-species, which differ clearly in many physical characteristics. Two centres of domestication of the pig lie in the range of the sub-species *Sus scrofa* scrofa, i.e. the European wild boar. These are the eastern Mediterranean region and the area south of the Baltic Sea. The third centre of domestication is in South-East Asia. Here, domestic pigs developed from the sub-species *Sus scrofa* vittatus, the Banded Pig. This now appears to be extinct.

Up to the eighteenth century, the life of the European domestic pig did not differ fundamentally from that of the wild pig. The conditions under which they were kept did not offer them any protection from inclement weather. They had mainly to forage for their own food in the forests, and were given only scraps. Occasionally, a wild boar would be driven into the enclosure to serve a sow. As a result, domestic pigs scarcely differed from wild pigs in conformation up to this time. They were long-legged, slim animals with an elongated head and a distinct ridge of bristles on the back. Around 1800, pigs were still slaughtered at 18 months of age in Germany; they weighed about 50 kg then.

Not until the end of the eighteenth century were pigs subjected to breeding programmes. This occurred first in England, and fulfilled three prerequisites:

- Incipient industrialisation increased wealth and thus promoted a greater demand for meat and fat.
- Increasing knowledge led to improved land husbandry and thus to higher yields. Pigs could now be fed better.
- England's extensive maritime trade led to pigs being brought back from East Asia, and then crossed with indigenous pigs. Neapolitan pigs were also introduced, which also originated in South-East Asia.

This resulted in early-maturing pigs which put on a lot of fat, but which were not very prolific. The short head with the concave nose line (saddle nose), inherited from the south-east Asian form, still exists today. The improved performance of the new type of pig is partly due to the fact that breeding animals with great differences in genetic make-up were taken from widely separated locations. But the enormous breeding achievement, which produced large, prolific pigs in England, should not be overlooked.

After 1860, these more robust pigs, which were more in line with the breeding target of the time, were also exported to Germany and were crossed with the unimproved landraces there. Up to the end of the post-war era, a large-framed, deep-bodied pig of the fat-pig type was bred in Germany, which was capable of utilising large quantities of local fodder (especially potatoes). Up to this time, improved landraces such as the Angeln Saddleback and the Schwäbisch–Hall and even the German Meadow as an unimproved land pig still had a place on the market. At the end of the 1950s, consumers' expectations changed in a short space of time. There was now a demand for tender, succulent meat with as little fat as possible. Buyers were prepared to pay more for the best cuts – ham, chops and fillet. So pigs were bred to produce as much meat as possible. This development led to long, lean pigs (with an extra pair of ribs) with distinct hams and sometimes prominent shoulders (four-ham pig).

A tendency to lay down a lot of meat is often associated with susceptibility to stress and changes in the colour of the meat. Furthermore, there is a link between meat quality and susceptibility to stress. Differences in the colour and quality of the meat are described by the designations PSE and DFD meat. P, S and E stand for pale, soft and exudative, while DFD means dark, firm and dry. It is true that, according to the quality requirements A of the West German meat safety law, PSE and DFD meat would have to be classed as poor-quality or even as unsuitable for human consumption, because it is watery and heavily discoloured or does not meet the standard for composition and keeping qualities. However, these requirements apparently cannot be enforced.

For some years it has been possible to identify animals susceptible to stress at an early stage. Young animals weighing about 20 kg are briefly anaesthetised with the drug halothane. The muscles of animals susceptible to stress cramp up under the anaesthetic. Such pigs are designated halothane-positive and are not used for breeding. Halothane-negative lines can thus be developed. Furthermore, there has been a change in consumer attitudes: it is being slowly recognised that fat is an essential aroma carrier, so a higher fat content results in tastier meat, which does not shrink during cooking. This means that, in future, another type of pig may be bred, one that is less susceptible to stress. It must be emphasised that meat quality depends on other factors as well, such as breed, age, sex, nutrition and husbandry methods.

The pigs kept in central Europe are predominantly white. In the case of partially pigmented breeds, either white lines were developed (e.g.

Piétrain), or selection was performed for less pigmentation (e.g. Angeln Saddleback). This trend is also the result of consumer expectations. It is true that there can now be no one who believes that black pigs have black meat, as was still assumed in 1924. Yet the consumer finds the black bristles left on the skin after slaughter repugnant. If the pigment is only in the upper layers of skin, the animal becomes white when treated with boiling water because these layers are removed when the bristles are being removed, if the temperature is right.

The number of pure-bred animals is lower in the case of pigs than for other livestock mammals. This is the result of the breeding methods used. Only some pure-bred animals are used in continuous pure-breeding. Normally, cross-breeding is used, i.e. suitable animals of different breeds are mated.

Almost 800 million pigs are kept world-wide. Centres of pig-keeping include China and neighbouring countries, Europe and North America. In large areas of the world, pigs are not kept for religious reasons. In Islam and Judaism, the pig is regarded as unclean and may not be eaten. Other regions, especially the tropics and subarctic areas, are not suitable for pig keeping for climatic reasons.

There is no other species of about the same size which is anywhere near so prolific as the pig. Sows are ready to breed at six months, have two litters a year and produce 8–14 piglets in each litter. This means that one breeding sow is sufficient to provide many pigs for slaughter. The result is a fast succession of generations and thus a broad basis for the selection of the best breeding animals. This permits fast developments in breeding and speedy reaction to changes in consumer preferences. Nevertheless, in pig breeding it is desirable to keep breeds which do not quite correspond to the current breeding target. It should not be forgotten that, after World War II, when other requirements were important, even the Piétrain pig nearly became extinct. Currently, attention is again becoming focused more on breeds of the improved landrace type.

No other livestock species has such a small number of remaining breeds as the pig. Some are kept in small numbers, so the four most common breeds in the former Federal Republic of Germany today account for 99.2% of herd book animals (**Table 13**). The situation is similar in Austria. While, in the former Federal Republic of Germany, the landrace predominates by far, and the improved pig is of only local importance, in Austria most brood sows belong to the Improved breed (**Table 14**). Only about one-third of brood sows are of the Landrace breed here.

Table 13. Numbers of herd book animals belonging to the individual pig breeds in the former Federal Republic of Germany.

Breed	1951		1968	1985	
	No.	%	%	No.	%
German Landrace (German Improved Land)	19,314	66.4	94.9	26,468	64.8
Piétrain	—	—	2.7	8,906	21.8
German Landrace B	—	—	—	3,429	8.4
German Improved (German White Improved)	1,878	6.5	1.3	1,701	4.2
Angeln Saddleback	3,880	13.3	0.8	48	0.1
Schwäbisch-Hall	2,859	9.8	0.1	50	0.1
German Meadow	492	1.7	0.1	—	—
Cornwall	406	1.4	—	—	—
Berkshire	280	1.0	—	—	—
Red and White	—	—	0.1	—	—
Duroc	—	—	—	93	0.2
Hampshire	—	—	—	144	0.4

Source: Pig Production 1985 by ADS *et al.*

Table 14. Numbers of herd book animals belonging to the individual breeds in Austria, 1978.

Breed	No.	%.
Improved	1,620	42
Landrace	1,270	33
Belgian Landrace	610	15
Piétrain	300	7
Other	120	3

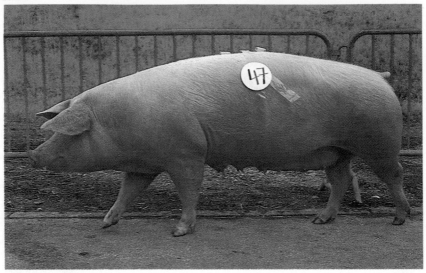

Landrace

Characteristics: Large. Long body. White bristles on a white skin. Lop ears. Long head with a slightly concave nose line. Mean size and weight of tested animals at the 1982 DLG show:

	Boar	Sow
Height at shoulder	86	80
Weight	312	273

Distribution: Distributed world-wide under various names.

Uses: Fast-growing. Good fatteners and good meat formation. High proportion of valuable cuts. Daily weight gains of about 820 g. Ready for slaughter at 100–110 kg live weight at 170 days. Prolific. Good rearers. Suitable as a female line for producing sows for cross-breeding.

Breed history: Developed at the end of the nineteenth century from a number of land strains, in particular the Marsh pig, by introducing the Yorkshire (Large White). At first they were not homogeneous in type or characteristics. Only at the start of this century did a uniform breeding plan emerge. As a result of changing consumer demands in the 1950s, the 'fat pig' of the old type was changed into a long, lighter 'meat pig' of the modern type. This was done via the Netherlands with pigs of Danish origin (Denmark had placed an export ban on those of its animals that best matched the new breeding target). This breed, which was known as the 'Improved German Land' in West Germany until the end of 1968, was given its present name of 'German Landrace' when the conformation was altered.

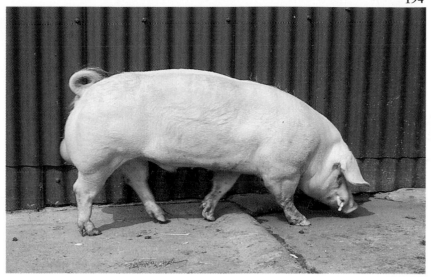

Landrace B, Belgian Landrace

Characteristics: Short, broad and stocky. White bristles on white skin. Relatively short lop ears. Well-defined hams. Mean size and weight of tested animals at the DLG show in 1982:

	Boar	Sow
Height at shoulder	81	79
Weight	287	270

Distribution: The former Federal Republic of Germany; no regional centre. In Belgium it is by far the most common breed. Austria.

Uses: Good fatteners. Very good meat yield. Good ratio of meat to fat. Well-muscled, broad hams. Good muscle formation on the back. Daily weight gains of 750 g. Finished at 95–100 kg live weight at 176 days on average. The meat is quite dark. High proportion of halothane-positive animals. Suitable as a male line for all-round cross-breeding and hybrid programmes.

Breed history: Developed in Belgium for extreme capacity to lay down meat by crossing the Piétrain with the local Land pig. Exported to West Germany from the start of the 1960s and kept as a pure breed there.

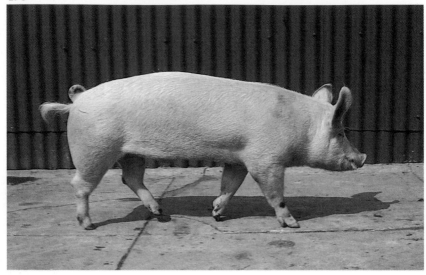

Improved

Characteristics: Large, of medium length. White bristles on white skin. Prick ears. Broad head. Concave nose line.

	Boar	Sow
Height at shoulder	85	80
Weight	320	280

Distribution: In the former Federal Republic of Germany there is only the closed breeding area of Ammerland near Oldenburg i.O. Otherwise there are only isolated breeders, although some have considerable numbers. The former German Democratic Republic. Austria. Switzerland. White pigs with prick ears occur in many countries under other names.

Uses: Fast-growing. Good-quality meat, average meat formation. Well-defined hams. Very good fodder utilisation. Daily weight gains of 840 g. Finished at 100–110 kg live weight at, on average, 162 days. Low susceptibility to stress. Prolific. Good rearers. Suitable for all-round cross-breeding and for producing sows for crossing.

Breed history: In the second half of the nineteenth century it was developed from the old German Marsh pig with the English Yorkshire (Large White) by displacement cross-breeding. Bred systematically for early maturity and fast growth. The name 'German White Improved' was coined shortly after the turn of the century. As it had been bred for meat yield from the early days, there was no significant change in the type when consumer preferences altered after the war. The Improved was kept in large numbers in the area which used to form the eastern part of Germany. Occasionally boars of other breeds are crossed with it in order to overcome the selection plateau that occurs as a result of the long breeding process.

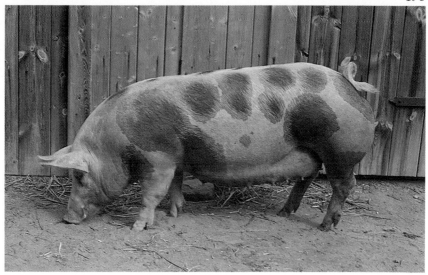

Piétrain

Characteristics: Medium-framed. Short, broad, deep body. Pure white, or white or light grey base colour with irregular patches of black or dark brown. Prominent broad shoulders and well-developed hams. Short prick ears. Average size and weight of tested animals at the 1982 DLG are as shown:

	Boar	Sow
Height at shoulder	80	76
Weight	277	266

Distribution: Many countries in Europe and elsewhere. In the former Federal Republic of Germany, mostly in the north.

Uses: Outstanding meat yield. Well-developed hams. Meaty shoulders (four–ham pig). Little fat. However, fodder utilisation is only moderate and they are highly susceptible to stress. Very high percentage of halothane-positive animals, which have been selected out for some time. Daily weight gains are around 700 g. The finished weight of 90–95 kg is achieved at about 180 days. Suitable as a male line for all-round crossing.

Breed history: At the end of World War I, pigs of the French Bayeux breed, which can be traced back to English Berkshires, are thought to have been brought to the region of Jodoegne in Belgium. At first, only one breeder kept these pigs in the small village of Piétrain, but soon there were many more in the area. For 30 years, these animals were kept by enthusiastic breeders without government support. By about 1930, higher returns were said to be achieved with these than with other pigs. In 1950 the breeders formed an association, which received state recognition in 1951.

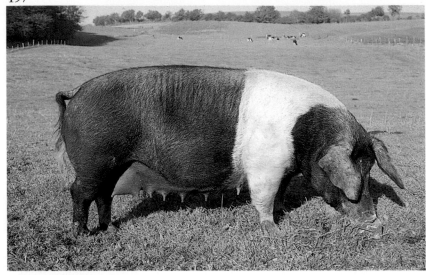

Angeln Saddleback

Characteristics: Large-framed. Deep body. Originally black with a white band around the forequarters. The rear half of the body is black. In view of the difficulties experienced in selling pigmented animals, there has been some selection for a greater area of white in recent years. Lop ears.

	Boar	Sow
Height at shoulder	92	84
Weight	350	300

Distribution: Schleswig–Holstein. Lower Saxony. Hungary. Czechoslovakia. South America. In the former German Democratic Republic, remnants are kept as a gene reserve.

Uses: Robust. Fast-growing. Daily weight gains are about 800 g. The meat-to-fat ratio has fallen to 1:0.55. Very prolific. Produce a lot of milk. Good mothers.

Breed history: The starting point was an unimproved black and white Land pig which was taken into herd book management by nine farmers in 1926. Subsequently, Wessex Saddlebacks from the UK were crossed into it. In 1937 it was recognised as a breed. After World War II it was much in demand as a fat-pig type; at that time over 60% of the selectively bred boars in Schleswig–Holstein belonged to this breed. Consumer tastes changed and the importance of the breed declined sharply. An attempt was made to bring it in line with the new breeding target by crossing in long, white boars of Dutch and Danish stock, and later also Piétrains. Some years ago, some Saddlebacks of the original type were imported from Hungary. These were the offspring of animals which had been exported to Hungary after World War II. Recently, some breeding animals were imported from the former East Germany. There are now only about five herd book businesses.

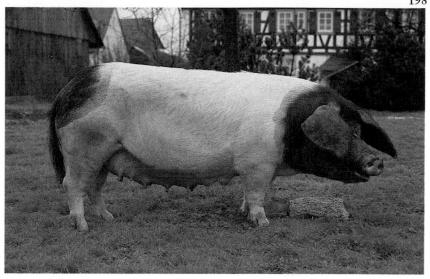

Schwäbisch–Hall

Characteristics: Large frame. Deep body. The head and neck are black, as are the tail (except for a white tip) and the rear of the upper thigh. The rest of the body is white. There is a grey band at the transition from black to white where there are white bristles on pigmented skin. Lop ears.

	Boar	Sow
Height at shoulder	90	80
Weight	350	280

Distribution: South Germany.
Uses: Hardy. Matures early. Exceedingly prolific. Sows are good mothers with plenty of milk. Recent carcase yields have been generally satisfactory. Outstanding meat quality. Piétrain crosses in particular make excellent meat pigs. Daily weight gains of 850–900 g. Long-lived.
Breed history: The 'Hall strain' has existed in Württemberg since the end of the eighteenth century. At the start of the nineteenth century, Chinese Masked pigs were crossed with it. In the second half of the last century there was random cross-breeding with Berkshires and other English breeds. A breed standard was established between 1925 and 1927. After the war, Angeln Saddlebacks were crossed with them. Around 1970 the breed society became dormant, as the breed could no longer meet consumer requirements. It has not been mentioned in the Annual Reports of the Association of German Pig Breeders since 1971. The Schwäbisch–Hall pig has been preserved by the efforts of a few committed breeders. Demand started increasing again in the early 1980s. In 1986 an Association of Breeders of the Schwäbisch–Hall Pig was reformed. There are now four herd book enterprises and about 30 breeders.

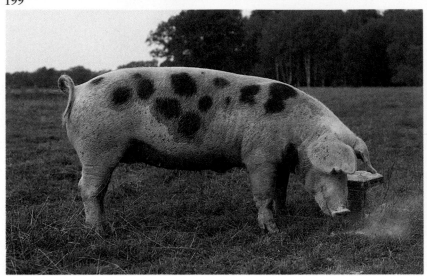

Bentheim Black and White

Characteristics: Medium-sized pig of the Land type. Irregular black spots on a white or light grey background. Elongated with a short pelvis. Lop ears.

	Boar	*Sow*
Height at shoulder	75	70
Weight	250	180

Distribution: The area of the county of Bentheim in Lower Saxony.

Uses: Robust, healthy, good rearing capacity with satisfactory fodder utilisation. Piglets mature early and grow fast. All halothane-negative. Finished fattened weight 90–100 kg.

Breed history: Descended from the old European Land pig. It was still widely distributed in western Lower Saxony after the war. At that time, the Angeln Saddleback was crossed into it. Piétrain boars have been used twice in the past

20 years. For almost 20 years from the start of the 1960s there was only one population near Bentheim. Recently, it has occasionally been crossed with other breeds, and additional holdings have been built up. It is also known as the 'German Black and White' or the 'Bentheim Land'.

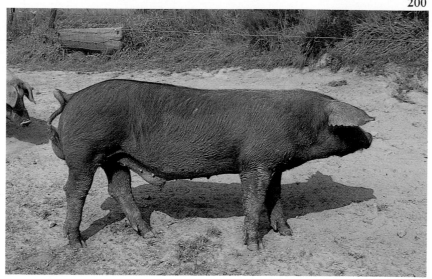

German Cornwall

Characteristics: Medium-sized. Black with no white markings. The head is of medium length and slightly concave. The lop ears are of medium length and point forwards. Long body. Slightly arched back line. Relatively short, fine legs. Deep chest. Voluminous belly. Deep flanks. Large bones.

	Boar	Sow
Height at shoulder	85	75–80
Weight	280–320	200–240

Distribution: The former Federal Republic of Germany. Hungary. The UK (known as the 'Large Black').
Uses: Hardy. Robust. Frugal. Grow fast. Placid temperament. Mature early. Good mothers. Long-lived. Suitable for keeping on pasture.
Breed history: The basic breed, which resembles the Large Black pig, was developed in England at the beginning of the nineteenth century using Chinese, Neapolitan and Portuguese pigs as well as native English pigs and also wild pigs. In 1896 the first pigs of this breed were exported to Germany and took their name from their region of origin, the county of Cornwall. They first appeared at a DLG show in 1901. After the war, breeding was concentrated mainly in Bavaria, but also in Hesse and Lower Saxony. In 1951 the Cornwalls accounted for 1% of herd book pigs in the former Federal Republic of Germany. Subsequently, the remaining holdings were rapidly disbanded, and now there are only isolated animals. In the former East Germany, Cornwalls were removed from the herd book in 1966. They were crossed into numerous other pig breeds, especially in eastern Europe.

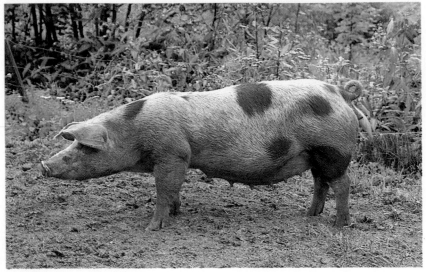

Baldinger Spotted

Characteristics: Similar to the Berkshire in conformation. Irregular black spots on a grey background.
Distribution: Around Donaueschingen. Today there are only remnants left.
Uses: They produced good fattening pigs in the earlier breeding programme. Mature early. Good fatteners.

Breed history: They were developed in the second half of the nineteenth century by cross-breeding Land pigs with Berkshires, and introducing Improved stock. As there were only small numbers, boars of the original breeds were crossed with them repeatedly. They never had more than regional significance and very few were left by the end of the 1920s.

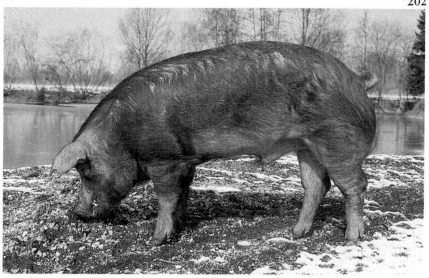

Duroc

Characteristics: Large frame. Mono-coloured, from light red to a rich reddish brown, occasionally with small, black spots. Small lop ears. Slightly concave nose line. Arched back.

	Boar	Sow
Height at shoulders	90	82
Weight	350	300

Distribution: North America. Europe. In the former Federal Republic of Germany there are only a few pure-bred holdings.

Uses: Robust. Good-natured. In the former Federal Republic of Germany they are used mainly in hybrid breeding programmes. Fast-growing. Finished at 100–110 kg live weight. Excellent mothers. The sows give a lot of milk. All animals are halothane-negative.

Breed history: The origins of this breed, which developed in the USA, are not entirely known. It is presumed to be descended from red pigs which were imported into Iowa from Guinea in 1849. Other ancestors of the Duroc include pigs brought to America by the Spanish conquerors, as well as red Spanish pigs which were brought to Kentucky in 1837. At first there were three red strains in the north east of the USA: Jersey Red, the Red Durocs of New York and the Red Berkshires of Connecticut, which were finally united as Duroc-Jerseys. There has been a breed standard since 1885.

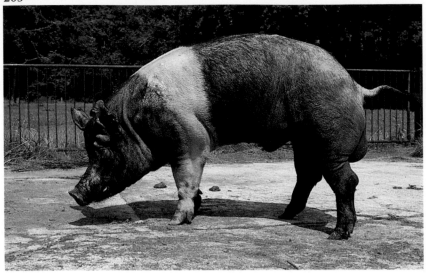

Hampshire

Characteristics: Medium-framed. The head and neck are black. The chest region and front legs are white. The rear half of the body is black. Long head with slightly dished snout. Relatively short legs. Prick ears.

	Boar	Sow
Height at shoulders	85	80
Weight	320	280

Distribution: North America. Europe. In the former West Germany, only a few agricultural businesses have pure-bred animals; these are mainly in Westphalia. It is the most common pig breed in the USA.

Uses: Prolific. Excellent mothers. In the former Federal Republic of Germany they are used mainly in hybrid breeding programmes. Almost all animals are halothane-negative.

Breed history: Derived from British Saddlebacks exported from the county of Hampshire to the USA in 1825. This breed was developed in Boone County in Kentucky, and was initially called the 'Thin Rind Hog', until the name was officially changed to Hampshire in 1904. There has been a breed society since 1893. It was introduced into West Germany a few years ago. It has not found very wide distribution as a pure breed there. In Switzerland, where this breed is more significant, American and English Hampshires are kept as separate breeds.

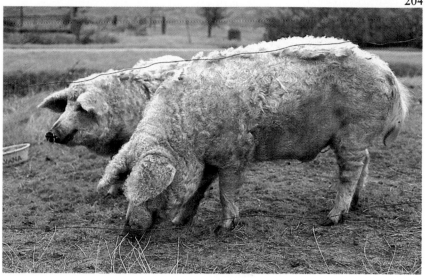

Mangalitza, Wool Pig

Characteristics: Large frame. The skin is slate grey. The bristles are brown, long and curly. Yellowish inner coat. Hooves, snout, eyelids and anus are black. The ears are of medium size and hang forwards. The back is of medium length and moderately arched. The pelvis is slightly sloping. Powerful limbs.

	Boar	Sow
Height at shoulders	85	75
Weight	350	300

Distribution: Hungary, Romania, Yugoslavia and other south-east European countries. In the former Federal Republic of Germany, only small holdings and isolated animals are used in agriculture.

Uses: Bacon pig. The thick coat enables it to withstand cold weather, but it can also tolerate high temperatures if there is a pool in which to wallow. Contented.

Small litters. In the former Federal Republic of Germany it is occasionally crossed with other breeds to produce pigs of primeval appearance.

Breed history: It is descended from the Serbian Sumadias pig. The Hungarian Mangalitza pig was developed by crossing this breed with the indigenous Bakonyer and the Szalonta in the middle of the nineteenth century. It was bred for good bacon yield.

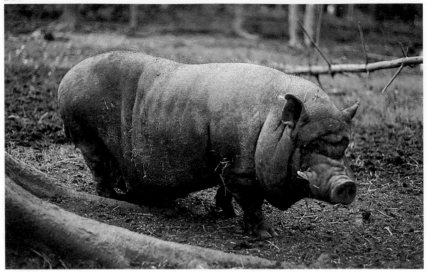

Pot-Bellied Pig

Characteristics: Small. Either all greyish black, or black and white. Short, very dished head. Small, pointed prick ears. Long, broad and deep body. Voluminous belly, which often touches the ground as the legs are very short. Relatively thick, often folded skin.

	Boar	Sow
Height at shoulders	50	40
Weight	60–70	50–60

Distribution: Vietnam. Europe. North America. Several breeds of pig of similar size are indigenous to China and other parts of South-East Asia. There is increasing interest in them in Europe because of their unusually high prolificacy.

Uses: Lively; may be very timid if they have little contact with people. In Europe they are not generally kept commercially, but as a hobby. Well-developed musculature. If they are not overfed they lay down little fat. Mature early. Large litters.

Breed history: Descended from the Banded pig, a South-East Asian variety of wild pig. It has long been a native landrace in Vietnam. The first animals came to Europe in 1866, for the opening of the zoological garden in Budapest. It was crossed with the Minnesota breeds, the Göttingen Mini-pig and the Mini-LEWE, a new breed in the former East Germany. Occasionally it is crossed with captive populations of wild pig.

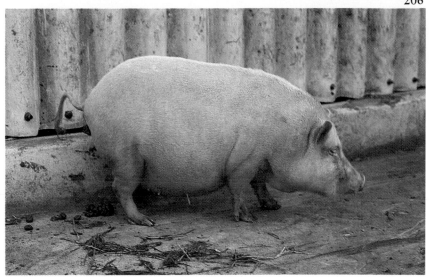

Göttingen Mini-Pig

Characteristics: Small pig with a saddlenose, a short snout and small prick ears. There are two lines. The somewhat heavier, coloured line includes black, brown and white animals as well as part-coloured ones. The lighter strain is unpigmented, and hence white. The boar and sow differ only slightly in size and weight.

	White line	Coloured line
Height at shoulder	35	38
Weight	34	45

Distribution: The former Federal Republic of Germany, the former Soviet Union, Israel, Japan and some central European states.
Uses: Used for experimental purposes in medical, veterinary and biological research. The mean litter size of older sows of the white line is about seven, and of the coloured line, about six.
Breed history: It was developed at the start of the 1960s at the University of Göttingen by crossing Minnesota Minipigs with Vietnamese Pot-Bellied pigs. Initially, pigmented animals were bred. As pure white animals were required by medical researchers, it was decided to cross domestic German Landrace pigs with part of the population, so there are now white and coloured lines. The breeding plan established was to combine the conformation and temperament of the Minnesota with the small size and prolificacy of the Pot-Bellied pig. Furthermore, the dominant white colouring of the domestic pig was required in the white line. The only breeding population continues to be located at the University of Göttingen.

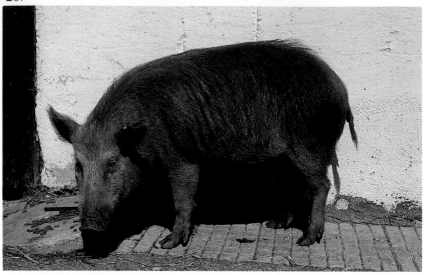

Munich Miniature Pig, Troll®

Characteristics: Dwarf pig. Small, straight back, well-proportioned belly line. All animals have white skin with varying hair colouring: reddish, black, or white background colour with black or brown spots. Most common colouring: light russet to whitish. The animals are relatively long-legged and have no pot belly. Prick ears are characteristic.

	Boar	Sow
Height at shoulders	43	43
Weight	35	32

Distribution: German-speaking countries, mainly the former Federal Republic.

Uses: Stress-resistant and CK-stable breed. Friendly nature, easily trained. Good intubation, normal vasoreactivity. Growth is severely reduced with feed dosing. Nuclear body-to-surface ratio equivalent by weight to that of man. Suitable for all human-equivalent tests on skin and other organs.

Breed history: The Munich Miniature pig was developed from the Hanford Miniature pig. The aim was to develop a manageable dwarf pig suitable for experimental work. In addition, the animals had to have a high resistance to bacteria, so that they could be kept without antibiotics. The so-called Columbian Portion pig, which is reared within the family unit by the natives, was crossed into the Hanford line. These small animals have a relatively high leucocyte density. After strict selection, mating the two original lines produced approximately the desired result in the sixteenth generation.

Rabbits

The domestic rabbit is descended from the wild rabbit (*Oryctolagus cuniculus*), which originally occurred mainly in south-west Europe, but did not occur in central Europe. Some 2000 years ago the Romans kept rabbits in enclosures, 'leporaria', for their meat. This method was later also used in France and England; it served to meet the desire for hunting. The first wild rabbits came to Germany around 1300, and they were kept on the island of Amrum. Real domestication was completed in the Middle Ages, initially in France, by keeping them in enclosures. The first books on this animal species also appeared here. Domestic rabbits were kept in Germany from the middle of the twelfth century, i.e. before the wild form. They were still kept very extensively in enclosures. Soon after the animals became domesticated, the first different colours and forms appeared. At the end of the eighteenth century there were already several breeds, including the Angora rabbit and animals with lop ears. Currently there are about 80 breeds with approximately 200 colour strains, which can be divided into five groups depending on size and hair length. In addition, there are breeds which do not fit into the normal classification, as well as new breeds.

Rabbits have a fairly long body. The neck is short, the head fairly long with long ears. Short tail, wool-covered and close to the body. Soft hair, varying in length. The individual breeds differ in colouring, size, form, and hair structure. There are dozens of different colours and colour combinations of white, grey, blue, yellow and black. Lop ears and Angora wool are prominent physical features of individual breeds. Adult rabbits weigh between 1 and 8 kg. They occur all over the world and are often feral.

Insofar as rabbits are not kept for pleasure, they are mainly kept for meat. All large and medium-sized breeds are suitable for meat, especially the New Zealand, Chinchilla, Large Silver, Viennese and Aries rabbits. The pelts of Short-haired (Rex rabbits) and Fox rabbits are made into furs. The hair is used in hatting. The wool of the Angora rabbit makes extremely soft, warm clothing. Rabbit dropppings are a valuable natural fertiliser in areas far from agriculture. The rabbit is one of the most frequently used animals for experiments. Dwarf rabbits are often kept as house pets, although it is often difficult to reconcile the different requirements of man and animal.

208

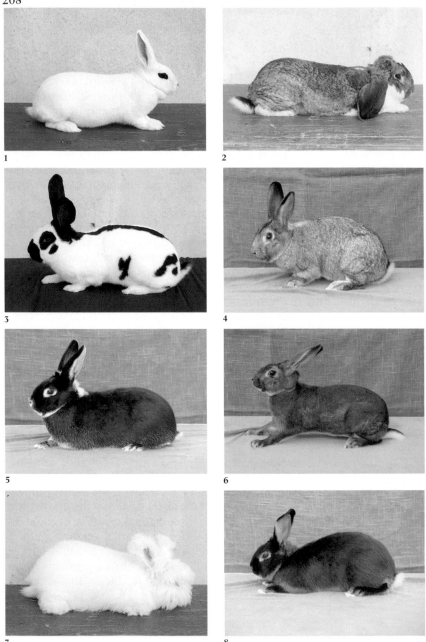

1

2

3

4

5

6

7

8

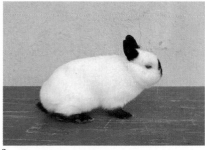

9

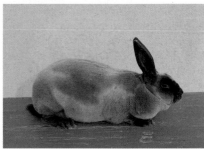

10

208 Rabbit species:
  1 White Hotot.
  2 German Aries.
  3 German Giant Spotted.
  4 Large Chinchilla.
  5 White Whiskered.
  6 Hare rabbit.
  7 Angora rabbit.
  8 Tan rabbit.
  9 Dwarf rabbit.
  10 Rex rabbit.

Poultry

An inability to fly, among many other features of domestication, is a characteristic of most poultry breeds. This flightlessness, which prevents the animals escaping easily, was achieved by reducing the size of the wing feathers and, in many cases, by increasing the bodyweight. Up to the end of the war, various species of poultry, in particular hens, geese and ducks, were found in every farmyard. This situation has now changed considerably. Specialisation and rationalisation have removed most poultry from the yard. Where there is still poultry in farmyards today, it is usually not for commercial reasons but because there is an emotional tie to individual species or certain breeds, i.e. they are for pleasure. In this case, it is not the highly productive breeds which are kept but, as is the case with the many other breeders of small animals, those which are less useful but have special features, or are decorative (their commercial value may also be considerable). When poultry were banned from the farmyard, the conditions in which most of them were kept also changed. They are increasingly kept on poultry farms; ducks, Muscovy ducks, geese and guinea fowl are still kept mainly in free-range conditions. Turkeys and broiler hens are kept in buildings and are thus less interesting to the enthusiast. Laying hens are kept almost exclusively in cages. The following figures give some idea of the situation: in 1982, 56% of the 42.8 million laying hens in the Federal Republic of Germany lived in holdings of at least 10,000 hens. They were distributed among 647 of the 302,000 businesses that have laying hens, i.e. less than 0.2% of them. These animals do not, however, belong to individual breeds but are hybrids, i.e. crossbred from lines of special breeds. Only in recent years has there been a slight trend away from battery cages and towards modified forms of enclosure rearing. The increase in productivity is impressive. In 1950, hens laid on average 120 eggs per year. The average yield of eggs per hen per year in 1983 was 255. Fatteners (broilers) achieve their finished weight of about 1500 g in less than 40 days after hatching. This weight is reached with very good feed utilisation. Broilers require less than 2 kg of feed for 1 kg of weight gain. Numbers of other types of poultry in the German-speaking countries are far below those of hens. Yet, for example, in the former Federal Republic of Germany, the demand for poultry meat can only be partly met. When keeping poultry, the origins of the wild form must not be forgotten. Even though some species have been kept in the temperate climate of central Europe for thousands, or at least hundreds, of years the basic behaviour and reactions of the wild form have not been lost. The species that were originally tropical, the hen and Muscovy duck, can suffer from frostbitten feet and, in the case of hens, the combs in severe weather. Waterfowl – geese, Chinese geese, ducks and Muscovy ducks – are only truly at home if they have access to water, not just for drinking but also for swimming. In the case of light breeds of hen and guinea fowl, it must be remembered that they can fly well enough to overcome some obstacles, therefore enclosures must be sufficiently high. For medium-weight and heavy breeds of hen, fences may be correspondingly lower. Waterfowl rarely cross fences although there are some exceptions such as broody Muscovy ducks and dwarf ducks. Male birds, especially turkeys, ganders and cocks, can be aggressive. Small children should be kept away from them, or be accompanied by an adult when approaching them. Sitting females and those with young will defend the eggs and chicks with surprising ferocity. Even if they do no harm to anyone, they can drive the unsuspecting away, which fulfils the biological purpose of this action.

Hens

Domestic hens are descended from the red jungle fowl (*Gallus gallus*) and possibly also from other species of the genus *Gallus*, which occur in the triangle formed by India, China and the Malaysian islands. The wild form was domesticated more than 3,000 years ago, and spread from India to China and later to almost all other parts of the world.

Most breeds have the following appearance: body carried horizontally, and approximately rectangular in shape. Large neck. Head with three featherless organs: the red comb on the crown, the pair of red wattles hanging from the base of the beak, and the white ear lobes under the eyes. The tail is broad, and in the cock contains long, sickle-shaped feathers. Hens vary considerably in shape, weight, colour and structure of the plumage and in the proportions of the individual parts of the body. Furthermore, there are breeds with feathered crests, naked necks, or no tail. The crowing of the cock is the most noticeable articulation. The weight of full-grown birds varies between 0.5 and 6 kg.

There are about 150 different breeds. They can be categorised as layers, broilers or fancy. Among the layers there are light and medium-weight breeds. The former include, among others, Leghorns and Italians, and medium-weights include Rhode Islands and Plymouth Rocks. The medium-weight breeds are also known as dual-purpose because they produce many eggs as well as a good meat yield. The main fatteners are Cochins, Brahmas and Orpingtons. The best layers and broilers do not belong to one breed; they are hybrids, mainly of the breeds mentioned. Some hybrid hens lay more than 300 eggs a year; hybrid broilers reach a finished weight of 1500 g in 40 days.

In addition to breeds in which the appearance is the breeding target, there are the fighting hens, which form another special type.

209

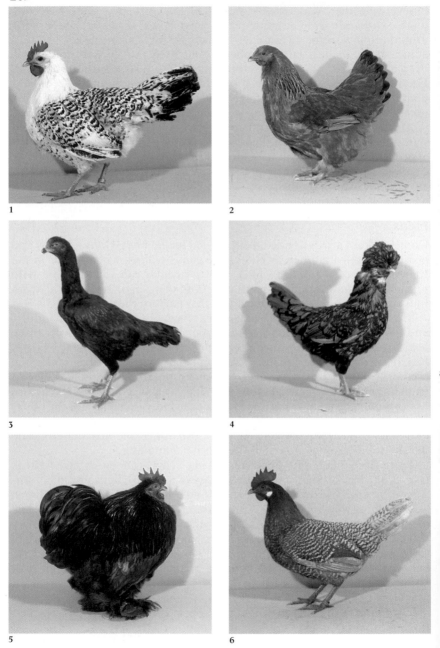

1

2

3

4

5

6

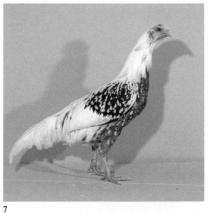

7

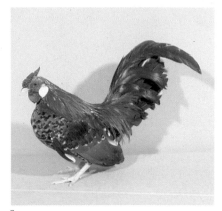

8

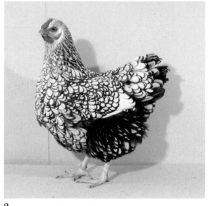

9

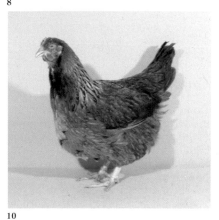

10

209 Hens:
  1 East Friesian Möwe.
  2 Dresden.
  3 Shamo fighter.
  4 Paduan.
  5 Dwarf Cochin.
  6 Friesian.
  7 Yokohama.
  8 Bantam.
  9 Wyandotte.
10 Welsumer.

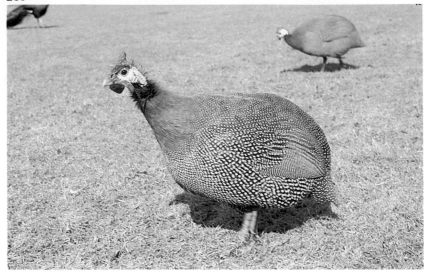

Guinea Fowl

Domesticated guinea fowl are descended from wild forms of the genus *Numida*, which live in the Savanna regions of Africa and are easily tamed. In Ancient Egypt the guinea fowl was a holy bird. About 2,000 years ago it was kept in Rome, where its meat was prized. Later, it spread across Europe, presumably via the Portuguese.

Its appearance can be described as follows: large, oval body. Tail points down. Short neck. Small, featherless head with a short, powerful beak. Helmet-like, horny protuberance on the head. Head white at the sides. Pale wattles. All feathers in the body plumage have several white 'pearls' on a dark background, sometimes in rows. The brownish flight feathers are mono-coloured, as is the shiny metallic blue neck ruff. The body plumage may be in various shades of blue, or even pure white. The sexes look almost alike. The cock differs from the hen by having a somewhat larger crest. Guinea fowl have a drawn-out, penetrating cry. They weigh 2–3 kg. The eggs are yellowish to brownish with a few darker speckles.

Domesticated guinea fowl are kept mainly in North Africa, France, Italy and Spain. Smaller numbers are kept in central Europe and in many other countries.

They have very tasty flesh and lay good eggs. The penetrating calls may indeed warn other birds in a poultry yard and scare off predators, but they can be so irritating to owners that guinea fowl are not a significant variety of livestock on farms. However, in some countries, specialised farms have been breeding improved guinea fowl in great numbers for some years. In a year the hen lays 100–150 eggs weighing 40–45 g each.

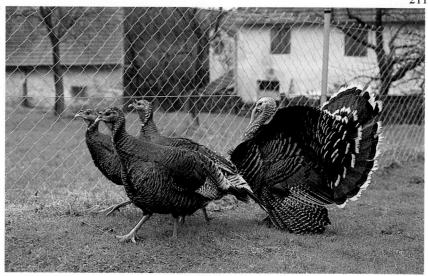

Turkeys

Domesticated turkeys are descended from the wild turkey (*Meleagris gallopavo*), of which several sub-species occur in North America. This was domesticated at least 2,000 years ago by native Americans. The turkey was brought to Europe in 1520 by Spanish seafarers. There are numerous breeds, which differ from the wild form in size, shape and colour. Selective breeding for well-developed breast musculature has been so successful that certain turkey strains can no longer mate due to the obstructive muscles. They are reproduced by artificial insemination.

Turkeys have a long, deep body and the breast is often very broad. The head and upper part of the neck have no feathers; the skin is blue and red. These parts of the body bear several fleshy protuberances. In addition to the wattles, there is a flap over the base of the beak. This is more pronounced in the cock than the hen, and becomes enlarged when he is excited. The tail of the cock contains numerous long, broad feathers, which are spread out fan-like in display behaviour. The plumage may be black, with or without a bronze sheen, blue, red, yellow and white. The most distinctive call of the cock is a loud, sudden gobbling. Cocks weigh 8–20 kg depending on the strain, and hens weigh 4–10 kg. The eggs are yellowish brown with dark brown spots.

Turkeys are kept all over the world but especially in North and Central America. They are being kept in increasing numbers in central Europe.

The meat is tasty and lean. The carcase has a high proportion of meat. The feathers too are used. In a year the hen lays up to 250 eggs weighing 70–100 g each.

Pigeons

The domestic dove (*Columba domestica*) is descended from the rock dove (*Columbia livia*), whose range extends from the Faroes, the coast of the UK, and the Iberian peninsula via the Mediterranean countries to India. There is evidence that there were tame doves in Egypt about 5000 years ago (Müller, 1978), and the Romans had strains of varying colours and varying uses. In central Europe there are illustrations of doves dating from the fifteenth century although they probably occurred there much earlier. In the eighteenth century there were many breeds which differed in shape, colour and behaviour. Breeding development in the second half of the nineteenth century was rather turbulent. The keeping of doves was given a boost by industrialisation. As the dove in its domesticated form is still able to fly, it can be kept in cities and industrial areas. For large sectors of the population it is therefore the last link with agriculture. The dove has long been a symbol of peace. As such it is often mentioned in the mythology of many cultures and religions.

Owing to the great variability in overall appearance and individual parts of the body resulting from domestication, it is not possible to give a description that is applicable to all breeds. The average conformation can be seen in the wild form, the rock dove, and the feral urban pigeon, and also in numerous breeds such as the carrier pigeon: relatively small head with a slender beak. Short neck. Stocky body with a well-defined breast and a large crop. Short legs. Tail of medium length. Fully grown doves weigh 300–1200 g.

The dove is the only domesticated species that has maintained pair-bonding. The clutch generally contains two eggs which are laid in a crude nest of twigs and stalks. Both partners sit on the eggs alternately. The incubation period is 17 days. The chicks are fed initially with 'crop milk', a secretion from glands in the head. Later they are given softened grain. A pair of doves has four to six broods per year. Doves reach an age of 12 or more years.

Doves are predominantly grain eaters. During growth and moulting and when rearing young, their food must have a particularly high protein content. Birds which have to perform well as flyers, however, require food rich in carbohydrate and fat. They also need minerals and trace elements as well as grit (small stones or particles of chalk) to help grind the food. In addition to water for drinking, doves need water for bathing especially when the weather is warm and when rearing young.

Dove breeds differ in body shape and structure, colour and markings of the plumage. The current official German Dove Standard contains 210 breeds and approximately 2,000 variations (Müller, 1978). This variety can only be considered by grouping them systematically. There are ten groups of dove breeds. The form doves (group I) include breeds with striking body and/or head shape. The tubenose doves (group II) have large tubercles at the base of the upper beak. Owing to their hen-like appearance, some breeds are grouped together as hen doves (group III). Crop doves (group IV) have the ability to inflate their crops far more than normal. The colour doves (group V) have striking colours and markings, without prominent body features (except feathered feet). Unlike most other breeds, drummer doves (group VI) do not coo when excited but emit a call which sounds like distant drumming. The structure doves (group VII) have special plumage features (curls, hoods, a tail resembling a peacock's 'fan', collars, etc.). All little gulls (group VIII) have a feather ruff (jabot) on the front of the neck, caused by a fold of skin. The tumblers (group IX) gained their name not from their appearance but from their typical behaviour: they plummet from a great height and turn somersaults as they fall. These are distinguished from the display doves (group X). The male of the latter type flies around the female in tight circles, clapping his wings loudly. Utility pigeons are classed as a separate group (also called carrier, homing or racing pigeons), and have their own organisation. Their ability to find their way home quickly from a great distance was utilised by man for thousands of years up to World War II. They were used to carry written messages in tiny capsules attached to the foot. Today, the breeding of homing pigeons is as much a hobby as that of keeping show birds. Furthermore, roast pigeon is a delicacy which is unfortunately rather rare in German restaurants, unlike in other countries.

1

2

3

4

5

6

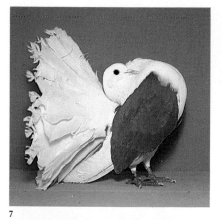

7

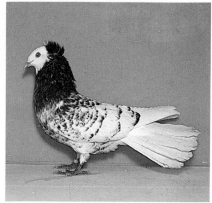

8

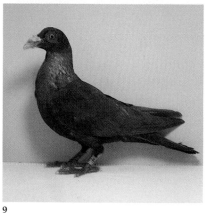

9

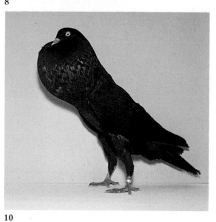

10

212 Pigeons:
1 Strasser.
2 German Show Dove.
3 King Dove.
4 Reversed-wing Pouter.
5 Nuremberg Lark.
6 German Dome-beaked
  Drummer.
7 Peacock.
8 Danzig High-flyer.
9 Steinheim Bagdette.
10 Steiger Pouter.

213

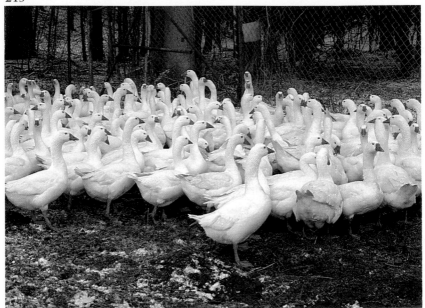

214

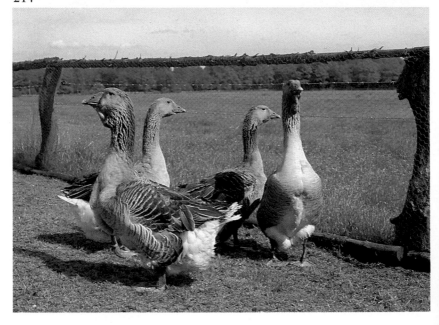

Domestic Geese

The domestic goose is descended from the Greylag goose (*Anser anser*), which, among other things, is used in north Germany for incubating eggs. Domestication began thousands of years ago; the Egyptians and Romans kept geese. There are numerous breeds which differ in size, colouring, and their performance as fatteners and layers. They may be crossed with Chinese geese.

The body is carried horizontally, or rising slightly towards the front. Long, elongated neck. Beak is set-on high and has a straight topline. Webbed feet. The birds may be white, grey or part-coloured. Ganders are only slightly larger than female birds. Some breeds have special features such as a dewlap on the throat or breast or long, twisted feathers. They weigh 5–12 kg.

Domestic geese occur almost all over the world. They are kept primarily in Europe, with the greater numbers being in eastern Europe.

They are used mainly for meat, fat and feathers. Abstruse forms of production include live plucking and force-feeding to obtain fat livers.

Fighting geese are regarded as a special form.

During a year a goose lays several clutches of 10–15 white eggs weighing 120–200 g each.

215

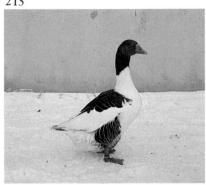

216

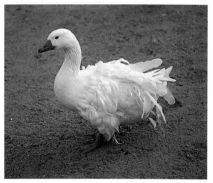

213–216 Various breeds of domestic geese: in the case of white domestic geese, it is usually difficult to determine the breed (**213**). Toulouse goose (**214**). Pomeranian goose (**215**), Curly goose (**216**).

Chinese Goose

The domesticated form is descended from the wild swan goose (*Anser cygnoides*), which occurs in Siberia and East Asia. It has long been kept as a domestic bird in China and Japan. In the eighteenth century it was brought from there to Europe. It has been changed relatively little by domestication. There are several breeds.

A slim, semi-upright body is typical. Long, swan-like neck. At the junction of the high beak, rounded at the front, and the forehead is the 'hump'. This is more noticeable in the gander than in the female, and is higher than the top of the head. There are pure white as well as grey-brown birds, which resemble the wild form in colour and shape. They typically have a broad, dark-brown stripe from the forehead, along the upper side of the neck to the top of the wings. The gander's call is a loud trumpeting. Female birds weigh about 4 kg and males about 5 kg.

They are kept mainly in central and eastern Asia, as well as central and northern Europe.

The Chinese goose withstands cold weather well. It is contented. The meat is tasty and succulent. Females lay 30–40 pure white eggs weighing about 120 g in each of one or two laying periods.

Domestic Ducks

The domestic duck is descended from the mallard (*Anas platyrhynchos*). Domestication began thousands of years ago, probably in China. Worldwide there are dozens of different duck breeds. In recent years there has been an increase in the number of birds which are crosses of domestic and wild ducks, living as wild ducks on areas of water near human habitation. These generally differ from the mallard in colour and usually also in size. Apart from Runners, the body is usually carried more or less horizontally. The beak is flat and rounded at the front. The head is narrow. Short legs. Webbed feet. Drakes are larger than females. In the coloured breeds, the drakes are recognisable by their more colourful plumage. Both sexes have a 'speculum' on the wings which is of shimmering blue with a white edging. In the drakes, the outer tail feathers form 'curls'; in the white breeds, this is the most noticeable sex characteristic, apart from the difference in size. They weigh 1–4 kg.

Domestic ducks are kept almost all over the world. The greatest numbers are kept in China and the USA.

There are table, laying and dual-purpose breeds; in addition there are numerous ornamental breeds. The specially fermented eggs which are particularly prized in China, and which we mistakenly regard as 'rotten', are duck eggs. Good layers produce 300 eggs per year weighing 40–80 g each. The down is another product that is much prized.

217 Chinese Goose.
218 Cayuga Duck.
219 Female Dwarf Duck.
220 Peking Land Duck (drake).
221 Male Dwarf Duck.

217

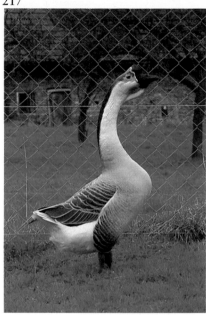

218

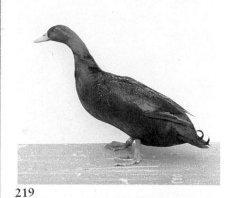

219

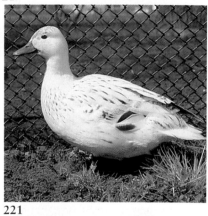

220

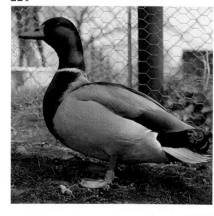

221

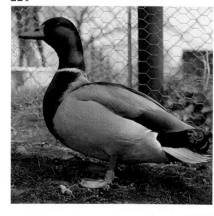

265

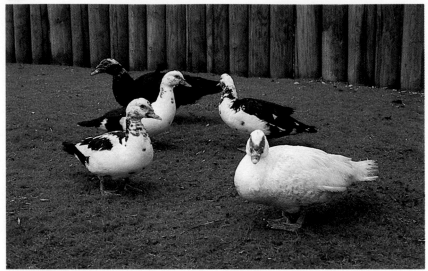

Muscovy Duck

The Muscovy Duck is descended from a Brazilian tree duck (*Cairina moschata*). When discovered by the Spanish conquerors at the beginning of the sixteenth century, it was already domesticated. Although it was brought to Europe shortly afterwards, it had little commercial significance here until quite recently. There are now a number of breeds. They can be crossed with the domestic duck but there may be difficulties owing to the different reproductive behaviour of the two species. Muscovy ducks are increasing in number.

The body is elongated and is carried horizontally. Short legs. The claws are curved and pointed. Webbed feet. Flat beak, hooked at the end. The area around the beak and the eyes has no feathers. Here there are prominent red fleshy protuberances which secrete a substance smelling of musk. The plumage is black (with white wing markings), white, yellow, dove-grey, or has patches of colour. The drake has no 'curls'. There is considerable sexual dimorphism: while the duck weighs only about 2.5 kg, the drake may weigh 5 kg. Unlike domestic ducks, which can sometimes make a lot of noise, Muscovy ducks can only hiss.

The Muscovy duck is kept in North and South America as well as in Europe. In the former Federal Republic of Germany there is no regional breeding centre.

It is sold as 'flying duck'. Muscovy ducks are lean and their meat is succulent and tasty. The carcases have a greater proportion of meat than the domestic duck. In a year a duck produces 100–150 eggs weighing 70–100 g each. Muscovy ducks are sensitive to very cold weather.

References

Anderegg, X. (1887), *Swiss Goats* (German), Verlag K.J. Wyss, Bern.

August, G. (1920), *Ancestry and Origins of Central European Domestic Goats* (German), Carl Winter's Universitätsbuchhandlung, Heidelberg.

Boessneck, J. (1983), *Domestication and Its Consequences* (German), Jb. Bayr. Akad. Wiss.

Borwick, R. (1948), *Keeping Donkeys* (German), Verlag Eugen Ulmer, Stuttgart.

Brem, G. (1982), *Principles of Pig Production* (German), Ferdinand Enke Verlag, Stuttgart.

Bundy, C. E. and R. V. Diggins (1970), *Swine Production*, 3rd Edn, Prentice–Hall, Englewood Cliffs, New Jersey.

Clausen, H. and E. J. Ipsen (1970), *Breeds of Agricultural Domestic Animals in Colour* (German), Mary Hahn Verlag, Berlin.

Comberg, G. (1980), *Theory of Stock-Breeding* (German), Verlag Eugen Ulmer, Stuttgart.

Comberg, G. (1984), *German Stock-Breeding in the 19th and 20th Centuries* (German), Verlag Eugen Ulmer, Stuttgart.

Comberg, G. *et al.* (1978), *Pig Breeding* (German), 8th Edn, Verlag Eugen Ulmer, Stuttgart.

Daniel, U. (1985), *Keeping a Cow* (German), Verlag Eugen Ulmer, Stuttgart.

Ernst, H. (1956), *Development of the Former Royal Lippe Senner Stud* (German), Med. Vet. Diss., Hanover.

Frahm, K. (1982), *Cattle Breeds* (German), Ferdinand Enke Verlag, Stuttgart.

Frey, O. (1984), *The Horses of Baden–Württemberg* (German), Franckh'sche Verlagsbuchhandlung, W. Keller, Stuttgart.

Friend, J. B. (1978), *Cattle of the World*, Blandford Press, Poole.

Gall, C. (1982), *Goat Breeding* (German), Verlag Eugen Ulmer, Stuttgart.

Geiger, J. (1939), *History of the Rottal Horse* (German), Werkdruckerei Robert Kleinert, Quakenbrück.

Glyn, R. and U. Bruns (1971), *The Big Book of Horse Breeds* (German), Albert Müller Verlag, Rüschlikon–Zürich.

Goodall, D. M. (1966), *Horses of the World* (German), Erich Hoffmann Verlag, Heidenheim.

Granz, E. (1984), *Animal Production* (German), 10th Edn, Verlag Paul Parey, Berlin and Hamburg.

Gravert, H–O., R. Wassmuth and J. H. Weniger (1979), *Introduction to the Breeding, Feeding and Keeping of Agricultural Livestock* (German), Verlag Paul Parey, Hamburg and Berlin.

Hammond, J., I. Johansson and F. Haring (1961), *Handbook of Animal Breeding*, Vol. 3 (German), Verlag Paul Parey, Hamburg and Berlin,

Haring, F. (1984), *Sheep Breeding* (German), 7th Edn, Verlag Eugen Ulmer, Stuttgart.

Hemmer, H. (1983), *Domestication*, Verlag F. Vieweg & Sohn, Brunswick, Wiesbaden.

Herre, W. and M. Röhrs (1973), *Domestic Animals – From the Zoological Point of View* (German), Gustav Fischer Verlag, Stuttgart.

Isenbart, H–H. and E. M. Bührer (1970), *The Kingdom of the Horse* (German), 3rd Edn, Verlag C. J. Bucher, Lucerne and Frankfurt am Main.

Kräusslich, H. (1981), *Cattle Breeding*

(German), 6th Edn, Verlag Eugen Ulmer, Stuttgart.

Löwe, H. and H. Meyer (1979), *The Breeding and Feeding of Horses* (German), 5th Edn, Verlag Eugen Ulmer, Stuttgart.

Müller, E. (1978), *The World of Racing Pigeons* (German), Verlag Oertel Spörer, Reutlingen.

Nachtsheim, H. (1936), *From Wild Animal to Domestic Animal* (German), Alfred Metzner Verlag, Berlin.

N. N. (1984), *German Poultry Breed Standard* (German), Verlag Jürgens, Germering.

Peitz, B. and L. Peitz (1985), *Keeping Hens* (German), Verlag Eugen Ulmer, Stuttgart.

Rieder, H. (1984), *Keeping Sheep* (German), Verlag Eugen Ulmer, Stuttgart.

Schaper, H. (1934), *The Small–Scale Goat Keeper* (German), Verlag J. Neumann, Neudamm.

Schley, P. (1985), *Rabbits* (German), Verlag Eugen Ulmer, Stuttgart.

Scholtyssek, S. and P. Doll (1978), *Useful and Decorative Poultry* (German), Verlag Eugen Ulmer, Stuttgart.

Scholtyssek, S., M. Grashorn, H. Vogt and R–M. Wegner (1987), *Poultry* (German), Verlag Eugen Ulmer, Stuttgart.

Schön, D. (1983), *Practical Horse Breeding. Sports Horses and Ponies* (German), Verlag Eugen Ulmer, Stuttgart.

Schwark, H–J., St. Jankowski and L. Veress (1981), *International Manual of Animal Production – Sheep* (German), VEB Deutscher Landwirtschaftsverlag, Berlin.

Schwintzer, I. (1987), *The Milk Sheep* (German), 6th Edn, Verlag Eugen Ulmer, Stuttgart.

Silver, C. (1981), *Horse Breeds of the World* (German), 2nd Edn, BLV Verlagsgesellschaft, Munich, Vienna, Zürich.

Smidt, D. (1982), *Animal Husbandry* (German), 5th Edn, Verlag Eugen Ulmer, Stuttgart.

Späth, H. and O. Thume (1986), *Keeping Goats* (German), Verlag Eugen Ulmer, Stuttgart.

Thein, P. *et al.* (1984), *Horse Manual* (German), BLV Verlagsgesellschaft, Munich, Vienna, Zürich.

Tylinek, E., Z. Samkova and E. Flade (1984), *The Big Horse Book* (German), Verlag Paul Parey, Berlin and Hamburg.

Uppenborn, W. (1970), *Keeping and Breeding Horses* (German), 3rd Edn, Verlag Bintz–Dohany, Offenbach a. M.

Wilsdorf, G. (1918), *Goat Breeding* (German), Verlagsbuchhandlung Paul Parey, Berlin.

Sources of illustrations

Association des Eleveurs de la Race Bovine Blanc–Bleu, Belge, page 70.
Edwards, J., *Wild Horse Research Farm*, Porterville, Ca., USA, page 222.
Euro Werbe- und Marketing GmbH, Hamburg, page 244.
Kamphausen, R., Mönchengladbach, page 128.
Medical Service, Munich, page 248.
Reinhard, H., *Heiligenkreuzsteinach*, page 263, at right.
Stauber, K., *Orpund*, pages 260 and 261.

All other illustrations by the author.

Index

Italic numbers indicate page with detailed description or illustration.